SKINHEADS, RASTAS & HIPPIES

ABOUT THE HALF THAT HAS NEVER BEEN TOLD

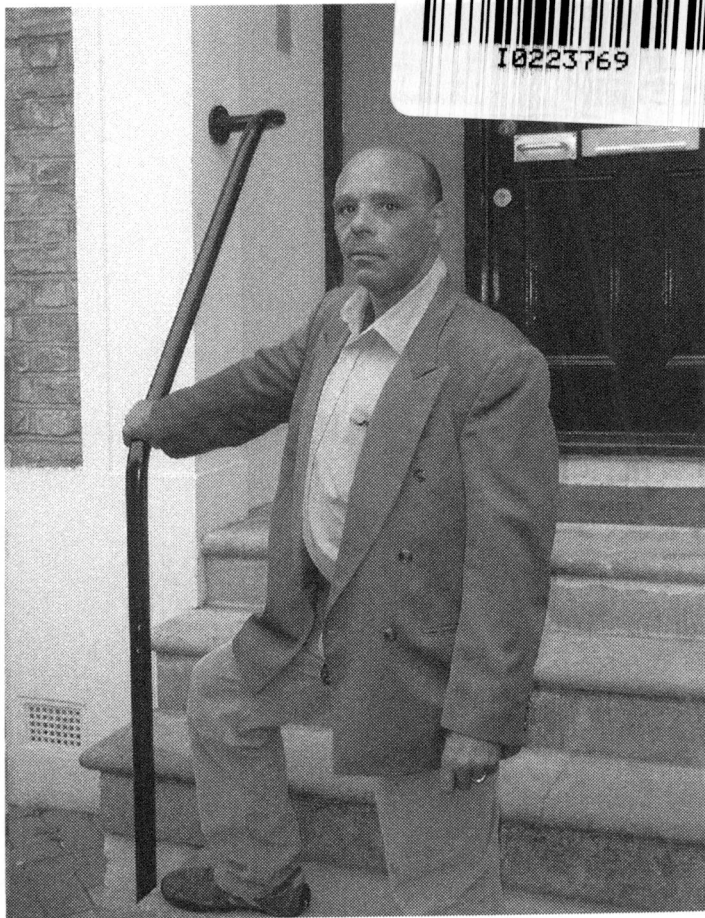

Published by:
Chipmunkapublishing
PO Box 6872
Brentwood
Essex
CM13 1ZT
United Kingdom

http://www.chipmunkapublishing.com

ISBN 978 1 84747 004 1

Skinheads, Rastas and Hippies

Now, now what's in a beard as you read it is B+ = B- add, which stops you from catching colds. With a beard you would see no chills what's in fashion is the medium size beard, which shows you are a man.

A beard is something that has been growing for a long time. If you don't have a beard it's because it makes you want to explore the art of shaving. But there are none that can say a beard is not sexy, yes, yes girls don't you know that a beard is prestige and a beard is really to make you stand out in a crowd.

Then again some people shave and find them self scared with shaving. Now the first one to break the act of love and shave would or should know there is no place like home coz it is fine with me.

When in Rome do as the Romans do and if you are in a company of people that don't well you are not expected to shave.

Now I wish you a home where you can meditate if you want to, now I wish you pleasant pleasure and true love. I say where there are Rasta's there is always peace and love and it does not matter if you're in the U.S.A or Australia, they are always the nicest and it does not matter what colour you are, you are always treated as brothers and sisters, but if you can't do as you should, you should move over for the children's sake.

So I had to say to a girl to tell you what I want to say, I want her to change not just to look like me but also to act like me.

I want her to talk like my soul that means just like the fit into my clothes. I say I want the girl to fit me like my soul so we can try on each other's soul; a soul is like a brother from the same mother or a sister. And when it comes to music it has to be soul music they call it soul music because no matter who you are the music sound just like you so that is good, and it is no big deal.

Now look what happened to the dead, the little actor that used to act your dream, would act your dream even when your dead, but it act to you but it is not you it is your soul your actor.

Ready steady go was not all it takes to win a race or one two three and never stop counting coz we've to find the right formula to win, you just can't turn up at ready steady go and except to win so keep on practicing and you could be a winner. Try and try and you could be a winner. I had dread locks but I had no religion nor did my brothers they say these days it is just a hair style, look how many people has long hair and no one wants to know why but as soon as they see someone with dread locks they want to know what does it mean.

Well it is only long hair but they look at it at face value and say it means religion, but it does not have to mean religion. I was a dread locks man and I had no religion nor did any of my brothers, it was just a hairstyle.

You may have heard on disc or records about what you heard on record but that is on record, records and real life is two different stories.

Now at a boy with an earring would you say he is gay, well it is the same with long hair there is nothing wrong. Now they talk, they are saying this must be the seven seal, they are saying how can this man be, but these things don't last long, most people go crazy over pop stars and film stars and say that they must be God but they come and go.

Now they are cutting their wrist and saying this must be God but these things don't last long coz kingdom rise and kingdoms fall all the time.

When you want to talk about something some people would walk over what you said and want you to go over and over even though they heard you the first time and they want you to keep talking to them, to make them feel important, and some think they would always get a reply.

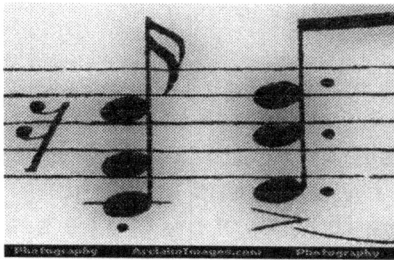

About the music some people are saying their music is the best but it is always like that, look at the start of the nineteen sixties, that was the start of the heavy rock music, some people said that kind of music was too heavy and up to date. Now they are saying the reggae has too much bass and is too heavy and they can't get used to it. Some of the studios say that the best reggae is recorded in the studio. But if you are looking for good heavy music the blues is it.

Stop from watching those rough televisions and listen to more music, coz these rough shows only make people violent, so make love not war and get your music out as they say music is the school of love. Keep the music that's what you would be more interested in anyway and that does not cause you much stress anyway.

After you have aired your point, some of us just walk over what they heard and want you to carry on talking but don't want to listen to what you have to say, they say that they heard it all before and they have no idea of what you said but want to put in their own meaning.

Hey they are opening a new Hospital, I wonder how much that would cost, but still the Rolling Stones keep on rolling without gathering any moss, maybe they should be up to different things like not letting childless couples have a say to people with children, so they should not have a say until they have their own.

To share a vision, well there is no one around here now so take off your security guard uniform and try on my new knitwear, put on my woolly hat, don't that take you back to your childhood wearing all these clothes that you was used to. There is no fault wearing these different clothes.

I know I try to wear as many clothes as possible. Earn money so get a job. There is no fault getting a job and getting rich coz there is no way you are going to get rich without a job.

I don't mind getting in a queue and one day you would get at the front of the queue coz there is always a queue and don't you know you could get that job and then you could make better plans and work until you are rich.

I don't want anyone to make a mistake and say it was he who told me that oh no.

Now while chatting to a girl the other day, we shared half of a bottle of lager. At first I thought she was new in town but after we got chatting I

7

found out that she knew me but I didn't know her, I looked her up and down she seems o.k. But the way this girl was talking you would say that I knew she said there is lots of girls in this town that knows me, she said I have a lot of budgie talking about me, budgie means people that know my name and talk about me a lot.

You know I did not think much about that but at one time I would be so pleased, she said they say they were my shadow and that got me excited but really I was not interested, and you know that some times I just can't make my mind up of girls, maybe because she wasn't dressed that good and I think appearance really makes the difference.

Look over a room and not moan, the way the floor is not so clean, right now room looks so untidy but don't worry about that don't you know there is lots of time to clean up and when you come in don't worry about the shit on your shoes if there is any.

Maybe you could keep your house spotless. Well I have never seen a spotless house, see I like my house lived in. I don't believe in spotless houses unless it is a brand new house or whom are you kidding. Yes I could not live in a spotless house that would mean a house without smell, a house where you can't do your own thing; oh no I would not be happy in one.

Could that be what they are teaching every time you wear your shirts, you wash them or take them to the cleaner but I think that is a thing of the past. If you have a bath you don't have to keep changing your clothes.

Sort some of this music that has been forgotten and give them to the kids. I am sure that if the singer was young it does not matter how long ago it was written as long as they were young at the time their music would not grey you coz the music keep its seal, so stay young even if the singer is old, that does not mean you would turn old and if they are dead their music would make you dead. Music and how it comes about is a very good love fire, it is electric and the same with camera.

Now listen to Beethoven love, how he sound as young as he was and there is no harm coz it was wired for sound and picture frozen forever so listen to old blue eyes Frank Sinatra without affecting you.

I am just saying better work than not to work just going around sorting out other people's troubles along the way, just sowing the seeds of love and harmony, if that is not good I don't know what is, just doing what a good Samarian would do.

You are getting used to me by now and you can't say that I am useless so I know you can like me coz I never give up on any of my friends coz I have learned to love and now it is love and harmony.

The best things are free so go to college and learn a trade they always say. You can have no regrets and you would be kind to yourself so that means you would be kind to others.

The morning chorus is staying cool, watch me go now, the reason we can get on with the right things to do, do you play the guitar like it's the only instrument and know how many instrument you could play, it is time we get it together and do more.

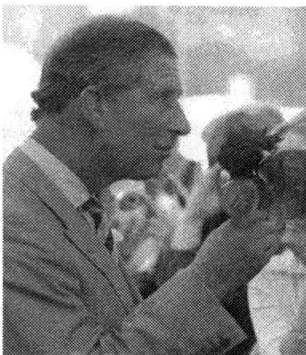

Can you imagine how much trouble it would cause someone if when someone has the same as a famous person, well it should, it would be no trouble, such as a name as Charles and they should not be shamed because they have the same name as a prince. Maybe you would call your son

Charles and watch him grow up to be someone even more than the Prince, a long shot but who knows.

At one time I said I would grow my hair until it reached down to the floor, but I only grew it down to my shoulder, which was quite long. Then I said to myself if I grow it any longer some people would say that I was dirty, but all the same, big up long hair.

Are you one of those artists that I have heard on music or in books that make you believe that they really are what they sing, can you say the blues man never told little fibs, the blues came in like the reggae. It was uptown blues are the best, and one from the east coast would say east coast blues are the best and the west coast would say theirs is the best, but now there is the same thing going on with the reggae, everyone is boasting that theirs is the best.

Maybe you could guess what stories they telling but it were hard to tell if they were coloured or white, but they were good storytellers. A day with my dad who they call Fred, but his name was also Jude, but he always get a word in, the other day they thought he said it all but he came on like he has not been told, with all new. His entire tale was heard; Jude would not lie down and kept adding to the day. He is the Captain Kirk of his day always up to date with what you would like to hear, such a sweet talking man, they say I am like him, I am his son.

So watch me go when I am ready to remember the good days that I had before were fun, counting on my fingers, sometimes, sometimes counting how much different music I had.

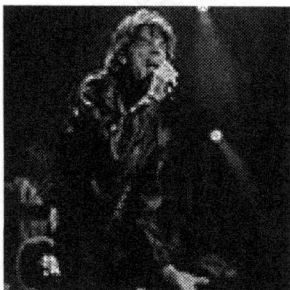

Sometimes the good rock music, how much of this how much of that, but I had to count more than once it was not like the police but the guy wanted to know how much rock music I had but every time he came to visit me he forget the time I told the guy that I don't only have reggae, I must have told over a hundred times but as I put on reggae he would say, haven't you got any rock, and he could not see why I would play reggae music and I would say some people must be born with the gift of getting me down even though I try and keep a nice selection of all different music, some people would like you to have all their selection but that was when I was younger.

Did you know that in my house there is no boss from outside but as I have to work I have many bosses telling me what to do at work so in your home no one should tell you what to do, what to wear, what to eat and what music you must play.

A friend said why are you so cool and you always do what you should, I said it is because the night is young and the frost is just settling on the grass and ready for the cold nights ahead and you know when the winter kiss, anything can happen, I am cool but how long would it last.

Oh you can't sit down like that you should be somewhere you can put your shoulder to the wheel and give a helping hand. Could you be there to help too because if it not hair it would be something else, hair that couldn't last forever, anything does not last forever but some is waiting for forever to surface anyway as me John would say.

Just because you are down that doesn't necessarily mean that you would always be down. I say not this time, even as I am rioting the same as you so look at this at an audit level, which is in the age of perfection so put your shoulder to the wheel.

Now give a helping hand but this time it's bumper-to-bumper and you say you would know who is fast or swift. Oh you look, I heard it all before but because it is you I don't mind hearing it again but they did not say because they was rich but if it was not a rich man then you would not even listen for a moment, so what are the poor man to do to be heard.

Just because I am a class A and not a beggar, can't you see I am working just like you and just like I always do. But as you know I have a lot to do, but it is never too much for me when it is you, I don't mind a bit of moaning and grumbling because we had good times too, all that I have done why would you see me like I did such a small sum, just like I never done much even though it is plain to see that I have done so much and I say there is a lot to do and keep helping some people get the weight of them.

I told one of my mates that when it comes to something you should know you are never there, here we are again do you know that song, oh what song, no I don't think it is in my house, but it is in the shops or I think I heard it in the cinema, but not wanting any one to know directly that they have that tune but it is nothing to be ashamed of, it is not you one that have that tune it might not be the only one with that tune. If you like that tune and someone say that tune is not good enough for you it should be thrown out, it does not matter and there is not supposed to be anyone telling you what tune to have and what you must not have.
Could you be in and out at the same time, they say this car is really good sunroof top but you are one of those that go by bus sometimes so you don't lose touch with the time so that if it get

banned from you, you would be in touch with the bus service.

Another time you say you are cheering me on and now you want to turn against me, it is not cool, when I say I am in love, that means I am in love and when I am in love but these days I don't coz my love never last long and I am always falling in love and I want my love to last forever.

Oh dear, now I have a very special little piece of love, a very special darling and I know we are going to miss and she is just enough for me. Wish you true love too.

Now hear this if that is not enough or is this too much well it looks as though it is, maybe they would search up on the hills and down in the valley and everywhere else that they have searched so far. No one said how much kids we are supposed to have, so it is not all lost. Look as my back is turned, they go and do the same thing again and again and again.

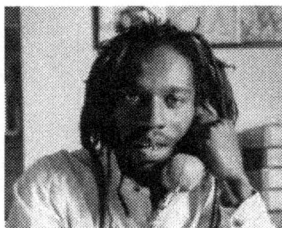

Where did you think I was looking, the hair again about too long get it cut, well this time we would have to make sure it does not as I ask kindly try and forget hair. Not like the last time as soon as my back was turned I could hear you mention something about dread locks. It couldn't have been such a little time ago this had happen but she come in exactly 10.20 and do the same and you act like you don't even know its your old friend John from Revelation, it's to make it easier for you to look like you have the same time as me. I never know what you would like so I am here to say it is not my way of setting up the work we have to do.

They say I am the loaf and other Johns are the slices, but I am telling you to let you know that I am not that easily replaced, that is what me, John, say and it's not too bad being John, as they say I am to look into the future. But as I am not easily replaced after all I am your friend. They may say Rasta's business is what John is about, no oh no, that's just one side; it is just my little sideshow. I am a lot more important than looking at Rasta's and things like that, much too important but I have time for it too.

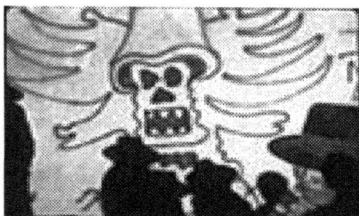

Is this your gang, I have been in a gang from morning so right now I have to be tough and I know how tough I am? Now they say we have no rules, and the pressure we are under did not last long anyway. Gang I soon would get over those days and the new gang look like mine, they say they have the same name; the gang has nearly the same name as some other gang.

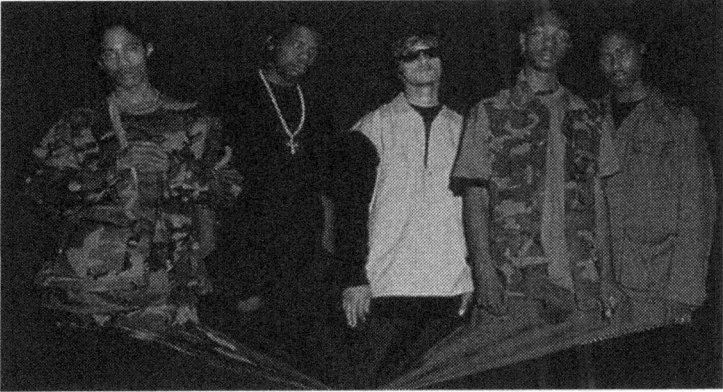

Their name is the Neutron Tribe a bit like tribes that were on television, a bit like the Rasta's twelve tribe of Israel and American tribes. We are one they say we are identical and there are forty-seven of us, but they say we are twins.

We follow the law and we are not violent or do we steal we are a good gang. A bit like the Skinheads we like to listen to the reggae music and also have the latest fashion and if anyone has any idea we would try them out, but we don't do anything wrong. We keep up the latest trend and the latest slang, they call me Johnny Reggae this gang is cool.

The girls and boys in this gang looks the same that is why we are forty-seven and we are not gay.

Now look how many laws there are and they don't even complain. Who would see you if you go into a charity shop and come out with some cheap item that would be good coz you done it for charity and that should please you, we are a bit like that. Oh yes a man of lots of different laws now you can go, the light has just changed but not just the law of the high way but we know a lots of laws to keep, there are lots of laws you don't need a police man to tell you, there are many laws another law, the law of Moses which is the original ten commandment. I don't say that they must do the same as me, but it would be good if they did.

Some people have not much money because they have no respect for the law yet they can get a grant of mercy [money], and I know you are young and know the right from wrong and what to do, that can't be so bad.

Well here you are again could you look into a crystal ball after the tune has in other ways when you are rich. Just because you know who is always there with the questions that doesn't mean you know all the answers.

Now look who is getting kicks out of snow it is not a big thing snow.

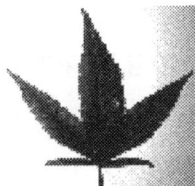

For there is so much for a husband and wife to do but don't say you do not smoke but where is the big deal, you can live without smoking but it is even better if you smoke at least two joints a day. Anyone can get on and don't even smoke anyway, even though they say it can relax you when you are nervous, I can see them banning and then bringing it back again to an extent of maybe even on the buses again.

What are they saying this one has no glory, but of course it wasn't too bad it looked all right to me, is there someone you know could show something like it, is to have children. Now they are telling me I should foster it out, you even say if it belongs to you it would be all right but because it did not, you would fight against a bit of smoking weed.

Now you are with me said to the one who wants my glory and they said they would walk in take my glory, of course you could not do it, it would not look good.

Why that guy doesn't have anything like or can't they find something like it and keep thinking it's up and not looking down. Now hear this since people has been dying they say there are seventeen billion in the past that we could find, even if we could assemble them there would be nowhere to put them. There wouldn't be enough space to build houses to keep all of them. Now a distant planet oh no it would take too long to get there about a billion years.

So the same someone said his plan should be tested so that we could spend money instead of looking to the stars in space we should look for many gaps in the past and we could spend lots of money going to these gaps time travel the people back in time where we could populate and live down there where there are less people down if any. We have to spend on great projects making time travel possible even if it took a hundred years or whatever it would be worth it.

You may ask me if I have been on a time travel well I say no but I know about it as in the past that I know that archers used to shoot their arrow in the air and it did not work so they tried to make the arrow thinner with no luck but it would be better if they tried to see the part in the television called the time base, which was made to bring the long time films up to date but that is only a fraction that I know about but to set the time base back in the past I don't know what they would do to be there when those films was recorded.

The time base but that is just giving a little light on the whole thing and the time base is a part of any television. It can bring up to date but I think it would be quicker than going to a distant planet.

If you can't get what you want you have to get what you need, there is a long gap between want have and need. Some go looking at fantasy ways like there is always a pot of gold at the end of every rainbow, some go gambling but some of us try and try all different ways so never stop trying coz one day you would get exactly what you want.

But once you find what you would want then you know you are there because you found so and make others happy and it so nice to have a family a few cats and a couple of dogs then only you should know what to do then and it would be nice to know that you got what you wanted. My idea is once you got make sure that you don't lose it back coz once you found, is much easier to lose it, be good and if you can't be good be careful.

Some of those people that was so sexy but when they found out who I was they did not know what they had to do to become my equal because it was rare because you said you have kissed well that's not a kiss it does not matter how outrageous you are.

Kiss you would know that is not a proper kiss coz only a French girl or man can kiss good and that is a fact, just like you wear shoes on your feet and hat on your head, well if it is not French you never had a kiss as you know French is the best like a stamp on a letter. Well their kiss is accurate like you did not know that what you have been getting was not kiss like they say that girl was not French. Well you know the difference between bread and butter and bread and margarine.

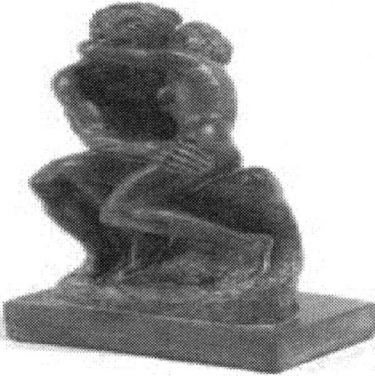

And now if you have a spare moment to tell you the French revolution was not in vain because they came with more for the cause of love they kiss so beautiful and that is the way, so if you want an engineer in kiss you can call me coz I have had experience with someone from France so anytime you call me oh yes send her to me and I might not be French but boys and girls I have a lot of practising you a few tips what I picked up from my tour, big up French kiss.

Look we should live in the future, exactly thirty seven years time there is going to be something happen it is said to dwarf everything that ever happened in history including Jesus and whoever you could think of it goes like this. They say there is going to be a great king sometime in the future he was black nearly everyone in the country was in favour of him been the king.

First he learned to play the piano and Beethoven was his favourite piece and he only played classical music, he also did art and soon got to paint great works in watercolours and oil. He was so powerful and had all new buildings build in his name, his people worship him and they started to say that it was his stars that filled the sky as far as I know.

At the time he came black and white was quite close so they did not mind him been black, they said that he came to make everything easier for us to live together and they said he took one look at religion and said anyone going to church had to stop and there should be no more churches black or white no one had to go to church and the people lived happily ever after.

It is one day but I took notice of what the fool told me about that king that there was like nothing before. He told the story so good I could almost believe that it would happen, he even had a name for him, he called him Hal, so much happened he was the greatest king ever even greater than any king of the twentieth century's kings, he made all the kings of the past look plain.

But really he was also plain even though he was black he would not let his people watch any film of the black actors of the twentieth century like Eddie Murphy or any others actors and all those reggae and funk he would not allow any one hear them coz people would say they were more than his people could do. They got on good with no reminder of the past music or film.

Look what they said about our mothers, mothers or just people that was in the Victorian days, look how they used to live, some of them said music in their days were evil some saw dancing and some saw high heel shoes, but this was a long time ago but can you see nothing for some people.

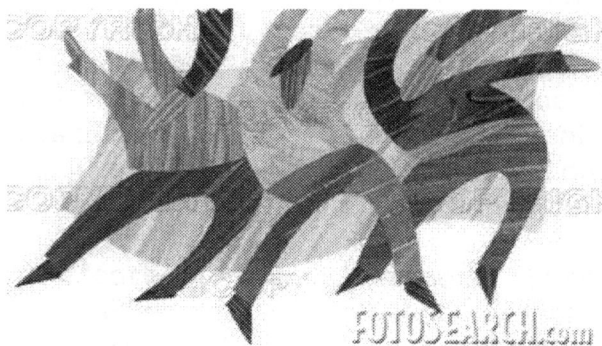

Now hear this man saying he does not like the reggae and they shouldn't play it so loud and look at another chap saying you shouldn't go skanking [dancing] you dance too wild and he did not dance [skank] like that in his days and did not see why the kids of today should.

Some people look at the lyrics and say why do they say this or say that when they know this kind of music is what the young people like because what some people of the past did not have, and their kind of music was not worth thinking about their songs, film or books. Now as before there are some people making up hymns like the past years. But this music is in demand and that's what the young wants to hear.

While some of the people say they should not sing such things are mislead because they don't use there common sense and hear the music as music, but they listen to it and then they say they are saying this and they are saying that, it does not matter what they say Jah, they would not wait to hear what else they said they would think it is wrong. Whatever they say is because they have friends and they sing what is in demand.

Can you remember when you were growing up and you would go to the record shop and buy what your mother wouldn't like you to buy. Say if you want a black girl your friends or mother would say go and buy records with a black girl singing and would help you to get a feel of it.

Some people can't see why anyone would sit down and listen to a load of dub; they lose their temper and say you should not listen to all those dubs.

They might be jealous or they are not in fashion, I am going to mention high heels, but these times are changing and it is different from those days.

Alright there are some of them say because they use material [from the Bible] they say they are singing these songs just because they believe in God but they just use material just to make their songs up to date and other singers use material just to prove they can do it also. So these writers keep using material like they believe in it, it is because they think they can make money because those songs always sell.

Lots of people only buy those kinds of records because it has words from the Bible. And again some of these people hate them because they say they are not the true religion that's what some folks say but can't they see the singer is having lots of fun as they make better and better music by hearing what you would like them to say, but the hymns writer of the eighteenth century also used material too, Big up song writers.

Isn't we all there, look at this how it use to be when I was living with one of my long time girl friends, we had two rooms one for the front room [the hall] and one for the bed room but I have just now looked back at it.

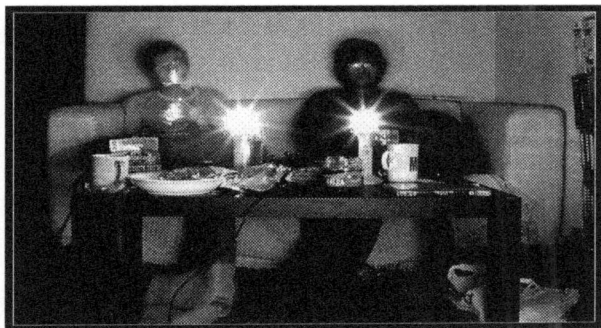

For two years we sat and watch telly at first it was not too bad but after a while it became impossible to stay with her, not that if it was someone else it would have been different it would have been the same coz we were young although she was not the first girlfriend.

So I am telling the tale how it might be with you one day or is it now. So I sat there day after day night after night just to be a good boyfriend but the more I tried the less successfully I was at living with her but we were young and it could have been anyone. I think it is always like that at first. To her I think that I was as good as gold now looking back I was perfect to her.

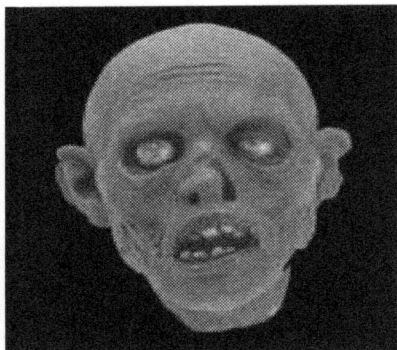

Night after night we sat watching telly and sitting in the same seat so I looked at myself sitting there in the same seat night after night and I felt like a dead man [Zombie] sitting there with her. Even though I would talk to her but it did not make a difference and words became fewer and fewer but it was not the talking it was just the same room.

I suppose that I am not the only one to feel that way in a first time love affair, but now that I look back at it, I bet my girl friend felt that way too.

So if you are like that now just sitting with the girlfriend don't feel too bad about that coz lots of people do that. I said it was not too bad coz life is not just a bed of roses is it. I think it was just a part of growing up a bit like teenage spots and those feelings do not last that long.

Now I don't feel bad about those days and I can see that it was better than being in prison but it was a little like that. At the time I had no confidence and I felt out of place but we kept each others company so if you are in the same situation don't worry it would stop just give it time and you and your partner would work it out.

Without a king you're your king, without a future you have to find your own. If anyone said you should have a king say you can do better without a king. They said the Rasta's king was very, very cold and had no remorse but I know that some people would act like he was good, good luck to those that think they can block the man coz he really was bad

It is hard to get though to some people coz they say if you have the hair you must be one, some are saying that every one legged man is Long John Silver, you said you have your picture with your dread locks in the picture and they say if anybody saw the picture they would say yes he is one of them so if you see any picture of dread locks just say it must be some sort of super star or some one good.

Now this day I said that I was to go on a diet to lose at least three stone in weight so I said what is the best method to try, but this was not the first time. This time I want to do it but I have almost tried everything from slimming biscuits to sugarless orange, so you have heard of cough care, foot care and a thousand of other elements of the national health service, so I am trying to see if I can get it on the health service.

If I can get it on the health service I know that I would get it for free, and they do so many different care services. I said that I would give them a telephone call some time in the evening just to see if I could have two weeks free health service slimming do.

But right this moment I am going to eat as much as I can eat before I go in that is if I could get the chance and then say bye, bye to greasy food. So far no luck so I am going to try the health farm and see what the nurse at the health farm can do. So wish me good luck for my care, what is wrong with going in care for a few weeks and when I come out I would be fit again for the road.

There are some people without value would see everything o.k. and as they see a little fault or someone cheeky talk they would break it to pieces a bit like Moses smashing the Ten Commandments, he smash them like they belong to him.

So some people start something and as they when someone got an idea that they know what the other person is doing and as soon as they think they got it now they said they could do it better but they do not say that they could do it without your lead, so they don't want to pay you for what you done so you smash it to pieces so that they could not find it again.

Sometimes I look at electricity and say to myself that it was just like that I say it was suppose to be a whole city with every thing like food and every thing that you could think of, you know electricity as in city but I say the first guy that invented it some one said they would kill him and take the glory so he smashed it to just a light bulb. So that should show other people that they should give other people credit for doing something.

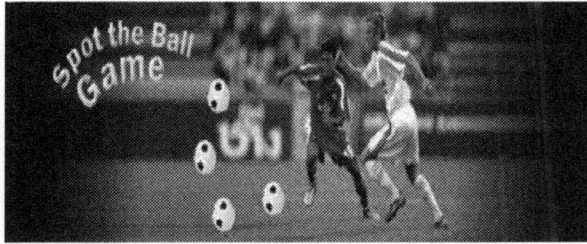

This morning I was far away in my thinking about some sound clash but I said to myself I wonder if I should go, coz there may be a fight and they are predicting that because the clash is between two of the local sound systems a bit like football when two local team meest, they usually have conflict but this was not football. This is in a disco dance hall or anywhere they play loud music.

You see you might have heard about sound clash that is when you don't go to the club to pick up girls on that day, on the sound clash day it is strictly music and the one who play the better of the two wins. There is not usually a fight as ordinary sound plays each other but this time it is a big occasion and when the music start any thing could happen.

The competition is where the first sound system play the first and then the second sound follow it up by playing a better record, they call it answering each other with music, so after one play something then the other answers with something twice as good then they go back to the other sound and they answers with something twice as good and so on and so on.

The winner wins a cup and is sound system champion. But my sound won the championship three years in a row and there seems to, as they are good to win this championship.

There has not been a fight at one of these sound clashes for ten years but the police said there might just be one today.
Rasta's give love all over the place so they should have a place in your garden, just like you see the black people and the Chinese the Indian and the white people so the same with the Rasta's men or women.

See the songs that they sing there is nothing wrong with them; they would do the same quality even if they did not sing about the Bible. But they choose to sing about the Bible and the do it good but even if they sing about something else they would do a good job too.

Anything Rasta's does they always does it better than other people. I once had a friend and his story was to talk about his budgie and every one that came round to our house when he was around he told them about, he told some good stories even though I don't think that his budgie was real, but the way he talk about this budgie you would think this budgie was so great.

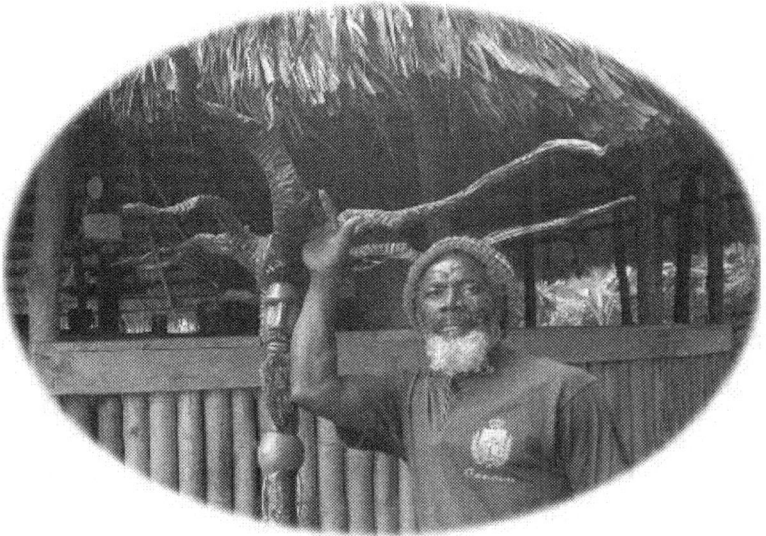

So some of the Rasta man talk about Jah and
they talk about it good sometimes I wonder if it
was real but that does not matter real or not it is
something to talk about, I think some of them are
like Delroy who was always talking about his
budgie but the stories that they talk about is very
easy to act out. I think that instead of going
around sad they can go round telling there stories
and if they did not tell these stories there would
be no reggae and that would be like Christmas
without Santa.

So my friend Delroy may be telling his budgie,
good luck to him. I wonder if you can sit and
watch telly when you got a Rasta man as a friend,
natter, natter and more natter. Don't believe

everything you hear when they are talking about Jah it is just to make up stories up after all it is well known to tell stories about a budgie so why not that.

I know that you don't like to hear them talking about Jah but when you get down to it, it does not mean anything, after all it is just words for real it is just stories and words nothing serous there is nothing wrong with stories.

And some of these singers follow each other [copy each other] in what they sing and they sing version of these songs to look like each other, they try to look serious but they can't fool anyone but they acted out each version like good story teller should. In pop they tell stories of love a lot of unreal story about love, and in reggae they tell lots of stories about Jah.

Who else could tell stories like a Rasta man, yes Rasta man is the best storyteller. In the future I can see them making stories like the ones Jesus has, stories like Jah made the cripple walk and don't forget Lazarus. Look how Jesus heal Lazarus so they can say Jah did something like that to make the stories more interested so there is lots of stories a Rasta man or Rasta women can make up stories to make their stories more interesting.

Oh dear, you've got your self a little piece of love, a very special darling yes and I know this is going to pass us and you were just enough for me, and it looks like we are going to miss, and this time if we miss when are we going to score again.

How much have you done since you have smoothed out all the kinks and how often do we have to iron out the creases out every thing is done except for a few more creases need ironing out and then that would be there, they always say that.

If you don't believe it even if you know it is a lie, there it must be something so small; it must be something that you owe or something that I owe. Now pretend that you believe and watch how much satisfaction comes in like that there is no right from wrong. Now can you ask the artist to tell you what it is, and what it could be but why ask question when they should know. Now check the time that it no you can't coz you don't want it. But there is lots of good times we had and everything here is right.

If you say what someone say get you down, you should know it could never hurt you, so sticks and stones may break your bones but don't you know that names could never hurt you.

Well look at this its only shallow water, not that it is in the news or on some big film but if its just talking in your own house you can say what you want. Did you know how much it cost me saying a little swear word, I think I am worth more than jail after jail. Feel free to talk coz sticks and stones may break your bones but names such and such, I wonder how much it would cost if it was on the television...

She says shut the window even if you are going out in the afternoon coz you could smell the smell of beer from the brewers and you should know that is what's pulling you to the pub.

Oh yes I am a can a day man myself you know, I must leave the bar now before I want more than one pint then it would be two, then it would be three then four and so on.

Oh not pies again with the same, yeah drop the filling; don't say it is pies again. Now is that the comb you used, when they said you were wrong after you gave all you could give. The comb isn't that always popping up.

Just as it was going good now for instance you would or might say I heard it all before as if it really has been heard. Then you heard the intro and go on like you heard it from the top to the very last drop, well you might say you ate the pie with no filling.

There are many nice things you do without noticing what some really cute thing a bit like when I am in bed laying listening to the bird's morning chorus. It is so nice to get up and brush your teeth with the morning chorus and some nice music playing in the background but not too loud, that is the champagne of life and it is not a bit unpleasant,

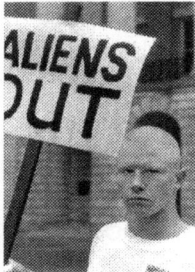

What did the radio say, video killed the radio star but books beat the lot coz you have perfect control over a book.

If you see me on a bad day you should know I had better days, smelling salt might do the trick for you to wake up, that is what I always do when I am feeling lazy and feel like no one loves you, well they do, just wake, everyone is loved over a hundred times over.

Do you go on like it could never happen to you like winning the lottery, well what about talking problem and keep out of trouble for a whole year, that would be like a big win. Everywhere you go you can find cash, they said the street of Japan is paved with gold, never mind if that is what they say and I know it is not but I think it is nice and it must be nice for them to say that.

Out of the entire sayings there is Hope, Faith and Charity, well hope is more for when Faith and Charity fail then hope would be like all three together so hope is the best of the three. I know what it's like to have hope, it brings you brand new aims but when charity becomes like hope and you know it is like oil to the motor. Wish you hoped coz it is a little bit extra.

On my mobile phone which has any functions but some people has problem with them, they just can't get it right but it is an improvement from the past years it is just technology in the making and I think this century we are going farer than we have gone before not just with phone but lots of improvement all round.

As will Rogers said in that herb man book it is something like that I was trying but drugs has got me lost well not lost but bewildered.

I say is not a big deal just picking up you tools of work and just go. But you have to watch out for the police. Don't you know to be rich means you never have to go to work, just sit around playing reggae music, rock music or even funk if you are a Skinhead, Rasta or baldheads if you are up to date with the good music, or go playing in Subway?

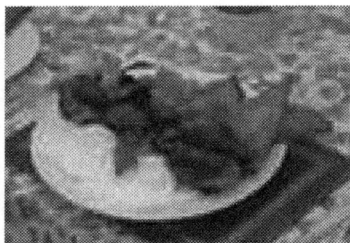

What I don't do on a hot day is sit around the house sizzling bacon, believe me it's no fun, believe me I have fried a lot of bacon and I have had enough of that for today.

I said going out side is better than staying in the house, don't you know? But what I do when I am out side you can have a lot of fun with that guitar. I don't care if not a coin fall in the hat coz it is just sport. Do you think you could do the same that was a day in the Subway? And now for my Broadway, don't you know if you stop with me, we could end up with a new lead.

Something like you would see somewhere else but I am here so stay with me, because its here is the hotspot yes it is here you don't have to be a Skinhead or a bald head or a mod, I think that I am the one and you are also the one yes it is so.

And you don't have to have a reason to celebrate any time with me. I am here to go anywhere you might want to go, and listen to the radio and there is the top twenty in the air you just curl with your wife get a few drinks and chill out. As they say for only a few hours a day you could find out how much you could do.

Now look round there is so much to do in the afternoon to have fun. I know this girl that is writing some new songs I wonder if she would write one for me. Not that it worries if she says could, she would not mind coz I can write my songs just as good. Now back to the book, the girl said this one that she is writing is wild and wicked, she says just wait until you hear it. But you must hear this one then the next one so they come, every one a winner, you win and sometimes I wish it were twenty million pounds or even more.

It is close to a good finding so we can work out lots of probability that may work out, what may happen? On any day, but don't drink, no don't drink for it may be any day now, I could give you the keys to my car and I don't want smashing it up. As I was saying it may be soon or it may be long time bet you would like a drink now, but you can find other places to go.

Oh come let me meet that girl again, oh how they say she is the nicest girl you could ever meet, but also the noisiest pot smoking, drum banging, almost as obstinate as a woman could ever be. So come quick, come before it's gone, in other words get it while it's hot.

You could meet the nicest girl but what is nice to you might not be nice to me. As some people of different race stick together, just like bird of a feather or like the leaves on a tree, let's make it so. Now let us make a giant recycle room where we can recycles all the dead and look how they would be separate after they are made back.

Now what we need is a giant recycle room with the dead of people of all different races, all different colours and make them back all separate but all brown can mix the people of different races. After the recycles chamber, you see where I wrote recycles peoples, to get all those people under one love which is like Uncle Ben brown rice, where you can see every grain separate, but these are people and they come out with everything like they suppose to have had, so they can choose, can you still see the melting pot after our generation pass over to the dead, what would the dead of before the recycle chamber react about us, bet they would think we are too posh, and we would be just like brown people after the recycle room ,we would be modern and might reject the dead of the generation before us.

Now look how I say our generation is not like them but we live and we are in peace and love. I bet the generation before us had their wine just like us but history failed to record it for us to see, it is the half that has never been told.

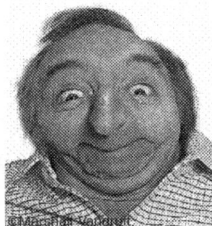

We could say we are the Coca Cola colour generation, and they are the Pepsi generation or something like it. And what if the dead of the past saw the 21st century all multi coloured and when the news reach them maybe they would wage war, and say we are the golden ones, and I know John that I am, would have to be there to coax them to do right. That is only if heaven call when I say John, I mean John of Revelation, the one that had to go into the future which is me.

But as love lives we would have to carry on sowing the seed of love and harmony, as we know that love lives and I am glad to be alive and I am glad to live in these times.

Lets stick together like birds of a feather, and big up Coca Cola. Stay alive and live up. As in guess whom is coming to dinner, the guy said, come and meet my family so be brave and get it on, or just sit together, and just vote if that's all you can do. But I must warn you soon most of the high places jobs will be given to blacks [coloured people] and that is a good thing, just like the sands.

Do your own thing, as a disc jockey put his music on every one say hooray, then the man does his own thing, about this tune I do play. Could that be the top spot what I have been looking for the past few years? One of those jobs where you are the most because you do your own thing.

While the disc jockey sits or stands playing his or her music, everyone loves a DJ and with rap and house music you can't go wrong. As he says from the top to the very last drop this tune I do play it makes me so excited. It makes me want to copy them sometimes. As you hear me you are not to be scared of me, hear the girl says you are not to hate me, you must try to give more love.
Well the wife Julie wasn't upset because she did not mind giving a little money to charity. I am telling you now, there is a man squeezing her toe, [when I said squeezing her toes I mean nagging for money]. They has caused her a lot of money problems, he has caused her lots of trouble.

First he asks for the time then he asked if she had any loose change, well some people also ask me for a little change now I think I should become a charity, you know what to lend any one money make me feel good, why well there was a friend that I once asked to give me some money, he gave me some money and I thanked, the next time I saw him he said go and laugh at me.

But do you know that if any one asks me for money it does not matter how many times I say to myself I would coz it makes me feel good and look richer. About you have your little friend and you keep giving them money like you are rich, coz you know you have a little dog to give small change to, I think that is so.

Hear me now, don't go on like you are not listening, it is not the first time they heard me. I know I have a lot to say so hear me now, now you are there you should not get into a state like that again, coz now we are friends. And then the chap said he would be good and would not even hurt an insect. So you might say you don't check that kind of things because it is new, and you may not fit the picture but you should be all right. Bring the ales in, and let's have some, you can drink but you see I am a driver.

You are not to hate if I cook you some nice steaks or something like that. Here we go shoulder to shoulder as I said before put your shoulder to the wheel and try not to hate and keep the wheel of love turning with lots of love. Hear me now that is that. When you have a friend it is nice but when someone comes between you and say they did this and they did that, you shouldn't blame them for whatever happens between you when an outsider influences it.

Didn't I treat you right that you would come back for more? But I told my lovers that does not mean I love you less than any of my lovers, no, not so.

Even though she said her mind was haunted and left a bit confused, but we did what we did in name of love. So I hope you are better now. Coz we are not a game we are meant to be good together.

Just the other day I had a hair cut, the wife said you should not have had that nice long hair cut. I say it was a dare when that person said cut your nice long hair off; I could have done it for charity. But I know I should not have that haircut, look how it would be long now, oh why oh why should some one be so unkind.

These men would do anything to deprive you so they could look in my pot and say you don't have salt even if there is salt in the pot. That is what a chef told me, but there are not a lot of those people, like there are about one thousand. So you just see the chef at united football ground cook for such and someone would say you don't have any salt, but how many people would look you for salt or should I say how many people would see little pork, look how many people would see pork, you would be surprise how many busy body would. I wonder if you could know what I would say.

I said to a girl the other night, about why you would get up this time of the night. You keep getting me up at all hours of the night when I like to just lay beside you and pretend that I am sleeping, coz no one could guess you had more than one drink last night as I put the bundle and put it in the dustbin.

The folk round here say is, get your scraps and boxes of a torn jigsaw and put it together and then one day you could get a job like that, putting pieces together and you could say you had a course putting bits and pieces together.

Bonfire night was when that ancient king was, it was something I learn in school, but I had to study, that was my most interesting lesson in school, the gun powder plot. But now you said you heard it all before now you are saying we should get a love nest, if that what we should get. How many times you look out of your garden and see that your garden is not the best, but you never look at your own until you see someone else's garden.

Look at that gates, it just needs a new coat of paint, and I don't want that gutter there at all, don't pretend the grass isn't always greener over next door wall. I don't really know but the way I have been in the last few weeks it must be, but not all the time. Right now I was looking at the commercial radio and I found that the products sell because it was on the radio, so here is my commercial break.

Who write the book of love, me wrote the book of love? Who else wrote the book of love, me wrote the book of love, who else wrote the book of love, well I think that how the song go you could call that a commercial break. I said now after that little rhyme I am going to have a can of Cola. Coz it is summer all the year round when I have cold drinks.

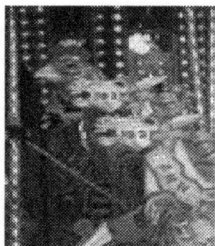

Isn't it funny how when you ask someone to scratch your back for you, you start by saying, go to the left a bit more, to the left a little more, to the right a bit down and a little more and a little up or a little to the right and just give up, wonder if that would break up marriages, just to sit and wait for the right back scratches to come along? Then you just give up and have a bath.

Bring a spare tyre when you go driving coz you might not have one when you go driving, because you never know what could happen cause 'a su'. [It is so]

In or out as you see some girl that I met said if she sees me talking to someone else, she has death vision, just to hear just one person talk to me it does not accept it. Why so didn't we have fun, what about you, and me I told her you don't have to be jealous? Oh yeah some of us know that I am a drop out, yes I have been a drop out for a long-time, well I not a drop out really.

But I have been hanging around and it looks like I am wasting time. You should know that good drop outs hang about smoking dope and not ever get a bad day, but when you hear of down and outs, they are even worse.

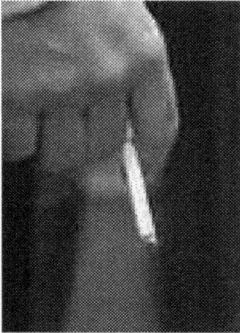

Sometimes I wonder if I would get back on my feet. So far the smoking seems to be all right. Now I am ripe again, big up dropouts. The truth is that you are trying to be wild and free, as you would like to be without problems, like sunshine after the rain, big up drop out, big up and have a better day. Or is it sunshine in the rain.

Can you see how much, right on and look how it recurs, at least have a good look. Look as I was saying to a good friend not knowing how she got to be my friend. At first we could not see each other's way, but look how now we see things like the same. Don't you know you can look back without getting angry?

Now take a second glance and I did a little show of what's on tonight, then you look again and it was corrupt, see if you could live with that. But that count is over coz you could fall apart if what you did was not wrong. This time it is good...my friend to keep saying maybe you want to go back in time and save what is down there, or even stop the big bang.

Hey, hey have you seen that new temple they are building up the road, they say it is a massive place. But I think we could do with a new temple and that's not all a big deal.

Come on now, don't you think we would need a new religion. Well do you believe in love at first sight, such could never in this modern day, with these days of divorces, but some people find the four-leafed clover?

But if a stranger comes up to you and say here is a million pounds, what would you do. Maybe you would kick your heels and score with a long love affair. But some people look for a magic formula for true love.

Now we have to look at love from two sides, it is not very easy to find true love but you could not be unlucky. I know that I am lucky. Aren't you a nice girl, well it would be better if I said aren't you a good girl. Don't you think you two are a good pair holding hands everywhere you go? It's not just in a sexual way, its just good friends.

Can you see where I was dear with that girl she wanted more of what I could not to give her? Even love is a story of men and women, and I am writing without taking sides coz I know you want a good read, black or white, coz I can't see what's the hassle fighting? So let love live. It's like I have being going out with you, you should get used to me by now my friend, you have become like an extra arm and that's a fact.

I want you to feel free to go to any party and just have fun with friends with nice clothes.

Mario's says to be married is equal to an extra pint. I don't know we are like jail or prison or sometimes like a holiday camp. It was so good to know that I got married and now has kids, and I am happy. I am feeling so nice, and right now there is no one like me.

The test of time is to know that who goes on common ground. Do you know the time when anyone greeted each other as 'Wotcha'. Well it still goes on, some new slang comes in, and slang goes out. Sometimes you just say a word that you just heard and you are the jock, the one that gets most of the girls.

There are many ways finding what is in the chart. There's a chart update every week, with the latest hit sound. Take "HI" for instance, it was done in the sixties when the hippies greeted each with hi or how. When we greet each other now we slap each other hand, or say something modern like you are the best, or say

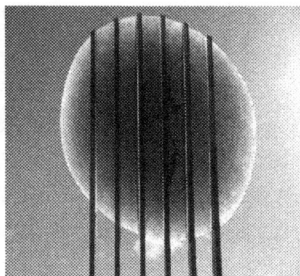

something like big up. As the generation goes on, the new generation pick up the latest slang, which was hand me down by the generation before.

Look how close you can go without losing in a football team, even the night matches are lit up so bright it's like sunshine when the floodlights are on.

Tell me your team could never lose and even if it did you would still support them especially if you are in a town where every one supports the same team, so they support the team not to be the odd one out.

You could not know how such fan lives, it is like religion how they follow each other. Some fans goes to see the match in the pouring rain; I know that they are fit. All the same the team I support I really would like to win the cup, some times I even go in the pouring rain.

When they score the winner, what a roar, and they have to roar as loud as the other fan does. That's not the case with me because I like football, but really I can do without. Oh yes. I can do without football. Not that I am not a good fan. I always play football with the wife and it makes me want to support my team even more.

Well we will see how many probabilities we have done, looking back. Oh by the way, have you or do you know that people in glass houses should not throw stones, well if you don't know, check it, don't you think that it is right.

Now look at those jolly fella's at out of bounds, do you think that pressure drove them there so they found that they had to go to an outer limits, after beating up a man or something like that anyway. Just so they can have their own way, you said the pressure is on and if someone said you can't do something or the other you would have to prove you could do it.

Same that you could get fat, really fat and you don't even take sugar. Now look someone said John saw what was coming, well you did not know how great I am, I am great not just of revelation, but hot of the shelf. Just like the best of the best in other words past where there are nowhere to go.

Now let's look at the matter for a while, let's see where John could go someone already said. These records was found, I was just getting excited but I am just as great anyway. But I know I am what to be done. Now let's make sure that it does not fall down on me, as the wise man say, build your castle on a rock.

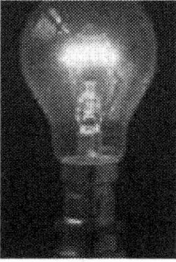

I am taking the wise man's seat for the day as John, who will smooth out every dream. Not too extra never too much; John Williams, yes of Revelation but just call me John, cream of the crops.

Now carry on, go on little drummer boy, I said one day while in Scotland, you can still hear the sound of the bagpipes and the fresh air on the Highlands, there was a mystery in the air. There could be no place like it, the smell of bread, and heather, you may say am I making this up. After hearing the sounds of bagpipes, just watch me sit in my room and listen to the sound of music, it was a good thing just like a stay in Scotland. Well I was not but the music made me want to be there. I can't wait any more I think I might walk it, so you take the low road and I take the high road and I reach bonnie Scotland before you.

Oh you don't need to decorate me today but I am not too bad, hear me out I am decent, but the way you talk to me it is like you don't know me anymore. What is the only thing I am doing on this ward is to dry out. But by the way you might find a thousand other reasons to say why I am here, I said I am not a drop out get it right, get it right, hear me out, don't pretend I am not nice and decent I said to her.

You say this is a nice place and you would take care of me for a few weeks while I dry out from my drinking alcohol, but now someone would try to add to my troubles, drinks and a thousand different reasons why I must drink.

Yes, oh yes said my friend why do you always give me not a good deal I don't know now said me, it is either you don't want to see me in front, and you would thank me if you knew me. One time you said you never knew me to have anything, but do you really know what you missed.

Every time I find I told some people it is like a gold rush, what some of those people know? It is a bit like baseball or cricket; they said they would like to get me out of the gold rush. Now back to the fact you said you never saw me with anything well you are wrong, well I said you don't know what you missed. I can honestly say there is nothing wrong with you over what you would do if you see me so filled with pride. Don't even think of it even though I would not give up my pleasure no not at all, I know I am right to do what I like to do, it does not even affect me anyway.

But by the way you are going on like I should owe you for a letter a week. I don't think that's a big deal so as she went through the door, and said' big up', now then what she left behind, I am just looking that it doesn't come back for them.

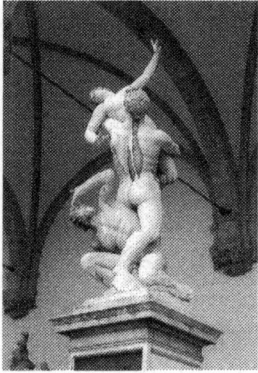

I could have said as she walks through the door but you might not know why I am glad it's not just me. Baby by the way, you said you have come to tell me the way you go, and asking how are you, and I don't want to fault you, I am so glad you are looking a little better now, such as you don't want too many guys to find fault, and say you don't fancy me coz I know you do.

But it is not like how it used to be, I have my house and don't want so many of you looking at my photo. You did not miss anything coz the photo did not look that good anyway, and someone say they would like to spoil it. I am always here to say, now the probe is off and I don't need a reason to do anything why because I am taught to do nearly every thing that I do, that is what school is for, but there are such things I do for my self such as sorting my money out, or women and sports and there is not much I don't know anyway.

Yes baby you seem to have your mind set on Orion, the gang leader, who is me, but by the way, you pretend you don't know how many of them there is. Well it look like the trend but you could say it is a lie but not one of those lies that you know, but a little lie is not even a lie at all when it is not important it does not matter. Even though it was not as great as it was suppose to be or could have been.

I said to my friends, as long as you keep putting me under pressure, you would not know whose foot print you are in. You would like to keep coming here, so every time you come you cover your track so you can keep coming, and it would be so easy to come if you just ask me. But instead you come saying you are this and you are that, just get it right and you won't be scared of me coz I am nice, and when I am friendly I give whoever a share so no one has to get a dirty deal.

If you can't dig tell them just pretend you don't know me. What can you achieve if you can't learn, there is lots of information that you can know about, and a great achievement ready to be found.

From the beginning of time men have been finding out how things work, there must have been many time an inventor started to make something of great importance and turn back without finishing what they started. So when someone starts to do something and finish whatever they did, they accomplish something that makes them more than the ones that did not work.

You say you don't know what I mean when I say are you for me or don't you really care about what I am saying. Well if you don't know this time why I am not beating round the bush. I could have been up in a big housing estate instead of been bumming around the streets if I had listened to what the laws said...

The guy with the bad influence should stop from going round doing bad and should be kinder and if you are perfect, who can stop you. If you are the Jock, no one can get in your way. Did you really know that the dream that someone is dreaming, you would have the same dream, and all the other dreams that any one has ever had. So love anyone for you would meet him or her in a dream, yes all each others dreams.

I know we have our own way too, but if you do wrong well wrong would follow you.

Can you remember those characters in those children comic books, did you see how they do prank and then pretend they are so good, I suppose that is alright but when it happens in real life then you know something is wrong.

Now look at it and say to yourself it's not and leave it up to me, I would get it sorted because you have the same plan as me. We are close, so instead of playing doctors and nurses just be careful it does not pay to try and be someone you are not, if you do, you would pay the consequences and learn to act when you have to do the right move.

Now can't you know why you can't see there is no need for it, it may be so easy to sort out, with a little practice you would just sort it out, or there must be a way out.

I don't say this would make a lot of difference to me coz I only say it to free up your minds, and mine and leave you with no stress.

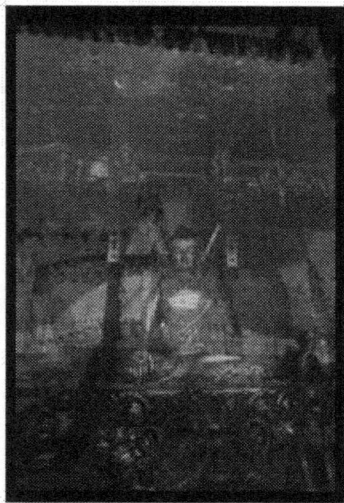

They say there is nothing wrong with going down and have a good pray, to even Lord Krishna and then laugh it off and if you don't indulge yourself, maybe one day you would come to pray to Jesus, the said powder potato would catch up now, Big up Buddha... Big up Jesus, Big up Lord Krishna, Big up Allah, and many more, Big up John. If you are just like one of mine, yes that is what I like to say,

Well could you come there every day since heaven knows how long, who never sinned as the good Lord said "If there is one amongst you without sin cast the first stone". Well see if it is not so and that it is tighter and see if it is not so.

When the act is on and they ask you how it is easiest to be active than to sit and count on your finger, just say you get a cheque for doing good. They say they get cheques for piss, when it is just a few of them take a whole company without any shame.

Now watch when they go down, a man must have his tolerance so he can earn his daily bread and get his achievement and pay for their days work without working too hard. And look, the same man they say he is their leader trying to tell me to shave, just saying he's not even a friend of mine, wasn't that right too for a man to go, about shave, what.

Hey here I am again with one of those ancients saying, well I would not do it today, but can you see the computer like the one that is on Star Trek, it is very good, well can you? Are you in control now?

Another exam over and seven to go, which is high-level exam result I must get? What if you know that you need to pass for a job and when you get there they say you need some more, exam, could you go on with it? You don't need a lot of sums to answer that at any level.

Mind what you say now a man said to me then he carried on talking in slang, like I had the wrong day. I say you can say what you like to me, and I won't get upset. I know that I would not be rude to the little man, that's in control, yes, oh yes. You are in control of whatever you say. But this day there is a group of people who are trying to say you can't say what you like, but you do know it is one-man, one vote. Isn't it the same with you, so did you have what and where it's at? It is time to be heard even if you are not in politics, be heard even if it is as a rock and roll deck star or someone who play music on the stage. There is nothing to be ashamed of, I can't remember where I heard that song, said the little man, but it was not really important coz you said the song was not important anyway. But any one that has come to spoil it and say you should know it's off.

They say not much happens in this house, but we have come to see about that, to make it easier. You say you want a better deal, but don't you know you must have the best deal as a guest. Lots of people like me know, so I would not look back here and now.

So what must I say if you like me, I like you too, now try not to remember that law someone begged and I had to cover a lot of hate on one hand and love on the other. There are many places to go and you would not be a fraud trying to be me with passport or whatever.

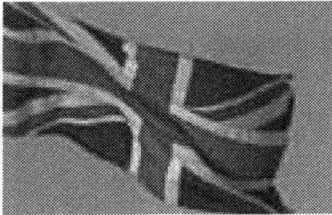

About you done this well, what's wrong didn't you think I could do it too, or is it only you could do something. Well you was not right I can also do it, long time ago the army was the only one that could do, but now the common people can have their say, and not so long ago you had to do for King and Country.

Now in these days you do what you do for you, make sure you vote you must have your say. Make sure you see your vote, you are not useless and gone to rust, oppressed maybe but not to lose in this world of opportunity and go from strength to strength and you get a better deal. With more money and things you can find lots of other sports.

Now I'll tell you about the time when I had so many things to do and there I was in prison with so much to do and no tool to do it. Not that I should be locked up, you know your crime and I know mine, not that I had a crime, coz they fitted me up. I spent all Christmas in jail with no one to visit me, but that was some time ago, As I got out

I said to myself I am never going back, and to this day I have never been back, I am here with you that big tough guy who has been in prison, that was a joke I am not big and tough and I was fitted up with crime I did not do.

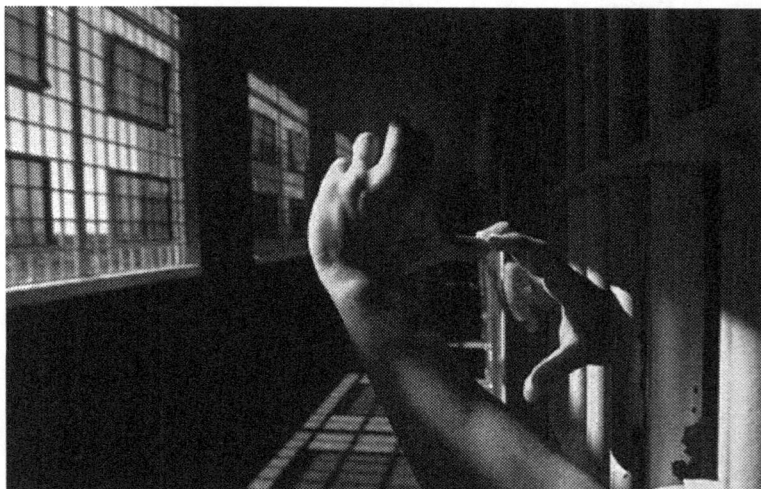

But I am the one that always fight for you, the one in your defence the one that you say stood ten feet tall, the one you should call your hero. Could you see me in jail with hardened criminals, what is wrong with prison is you get a bad name when you come out and the children should be taught that it does not happen to them. Well I am thinking of joining a gang, well again I am in a gang, a gang of punk boys calling themselves the Neutron Tribes. Not the tribes that has been on television but a new name for the gang, or not the Zulu tribes.

Now all I have to do is adjust my belt, or roll up my sleeve and the other gang would run off to hide but to wait for me to go so they could come back after I have gone home, you must stand close to me, but really I am like a mouse that would not hurt anyone.

Oh, there is not anything you could do to separate us; I say you are so close you are an extra arm to me. Now let me tell you how it was this time last week, well I am not sure if this love affair would last, but at the moment it looks like it could last for a long time, and we know that it is not just money, no it's not money, hooray, it's not money it's love, but its money too.

After hearing this you would not know if you should laugh or cry, oh yes, you would not know if you should laugh or cry that's what you say now. Wait now it's like a clown in a circus, you said it was sad, and I said it was like one of those hot numbers, clowns is supposed to be happy and happy they are. It was so much fun, after what they were the best stunt actor, but much better than these actor these days.

You are sitting pretty waiting to see which one is more like the picture; painted by one of those artists, when you look at it you just like the picture.

Well this is a show, now we are at one of those

towns where the entire houses look the same on the street in that town, now look one of them has changed the front door, what a rebel. Pin the tail on the donkey, for it is hot and you know it is an illusion. Now you are saying you heard it too look at it very long and it goes like it for any weather or any situation now look at how some tune sounds the same.

The Christian man would say Jesus would pin the tail on the donkey, some of them would say Jah would pin the tail on the donkey, the Muslim would say Allah would pin the tail on the donkey, and so on.

Which one is right, which one is going to do it? Who would know to a child, and would the child know who is supposed to pin the tail on the donkey. Well really you should pin the tail on the donkey, or if heaven calls well me John Williams [John of Revelation] should pin the tail on the donkey. Would them the child if he or she picked Jesus or Allah, whatever one they picked. You could pretend you did not see, so pin the tail on the donkey.

Now if you heard a song that you heard years ago and now the younger ones just heard it for the first time would you spoil their fun by saying it is not as good as the one you heard, you passed that so can they and don't you know that the new one would be more anyway.

Now can you see what I am saying about how some people get jealous of somebody else's hair, and some of them look at shoes, some of them look at clothes, some of them look at hats. In other words some of them comb hair, some look at shoes, some of them even food.

What I'm trying to say what if the man had long hair or would that matter and even if he wears hats, and would someone wear a hat well it must be to hide their grey, or is it practice for when you are grey, anyone can wear hats, big up hat wearers.

What I am trying to say, so what if a man has long hair, or what would it matter if he wears a hat, would I get red hot over that, well quite the opposite. I thought it would be nice to do what you like, then again if a man smokes there some people would say why do you smoke spliff, you could go without. And know that once you started you can get addicted, and once you are addicted you can't stop that easily.

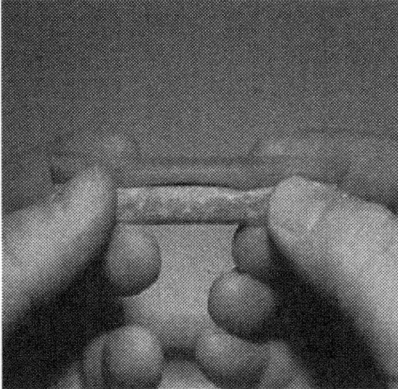

He wanted to touch everything, well not all the

tunes but nearly all the tunes. They kept on singing something like they sing the same kind of songs, but they were good. I could not make out if it's the music or whatever it was, but you could hear the reggae beat in their languages as they talk [not rap] and all they knew is why do you have so much fun. [Listen to music]. I would play the best tune and see if the dear boy knows that I put him with the girl if they would behave coz they need to get their own music if they needed it.

Now hear an Islam said you should look all around for a hypocrite and then he said the Christian religion is corrupt without looking at the Christian religion. Oh yes that's how the game is like football, each team thinks they are the best, and that is how it is done and that's the way it should be. Don't you think my team is the best, or are you not going to join me?

They say my religion is the best and they follow it with third eyes half open looking for something better. Well I wonder if it is so, or have they not got anything better to do. Maybe they had nothing else to do so they picked up religion to help, their day goes smooth and every religion is a winner when it is new, but don't you think you should be able to change who you pray to when you want to change?

Can't you get that the end product is always a

game, but when it comes to money that is not a joke because most of us like money, well I like lots of money. Can't you see the Christian hymns were written by someone just to catch the choirgirl? Maybe the first hymns did not win her so he did another and another until she get one and then he would be alright, and he could stop writing hymns.

I wonder who is going to win the cup or who is going to be champion in the football championship. I look at religion as a place of spending time until you find a better place to go and that is all right with me. Just a smile and I know she is mine; well that's what I say.

Oh how the day was rainy and what kind of mood I was in, rainy days always gets me down. Here I go, why don't you fuck off and stop fucking up my rainy day, I might be angry now, but it won't last now, it's just another rainy day so I would not take out my anger on any one at all.

There we are again you want to tell me that it is about time I have a pint even though you know that I have just come out from hospital after having a dry out, oh yes the temptation is strong to give up drinking. Anyway I can't drink any more lager coz I am also trying to keep my driving license clear. He is telling me Lear, but I know Lear would be remembered as one of the greatest kings of all time even though you know King Lear was not really a king.

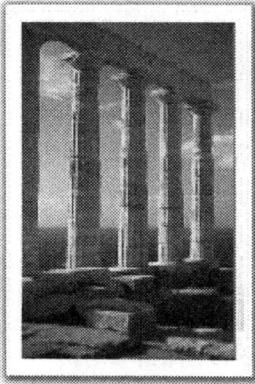

One day all the kings would be forgotten and it would be written as and remembered as story as in Greek mythology, they had so many great Gods and they are now looked on as stories. Maybe Charles the others and I will be forgotten one day and we could look at them as stories.

All the roads are marked correctly so as you know there is no need to get lost, and the danger of it is if you drink and drive, they say drink is worst than smoking.

Now, now sleepy head you must wake up, it would make a change for you to be up early, not just because you, yes you, you are not respected coz you never get up on time, that is you have never had a time to get up, coz you don't work. Get yourself together coz you are respected, coz you are someone.

You should not listen to all you hear as you know what real and what is make belief is you can see it plain as a kiss. Our love and affection is thrown to rest on the sea bed, we have lost most of the time we had that come in like we are so close, and now it is ready to surface. Let us try even though we can find that we don't have a lot, we can find without it coz it is so, it is to find.

We are not mean, we do not love every minute of it, Wonder if the song is right, and you are supposed to find it and be happy. You can't find such love that makes you have to re-load such love for a person like you, and yet you are even more than just the head of your house.

How some days drag when it is raining, now don't you know when the rain is over there is always sunshine again. It is always nice to know that there'll always be sunshine after the rain.

How many times can you watch the same video or how many times can you do something that you do not want to do, if you do the wrong thing and you are always wrong and never right, well there is always a light at the end of the tunnel. Do you like how I put it sunshine the after the rain or sunshine in the rain.

I really meant to say even if you are always down, it is not that you would get over today, wait for a better day, a better day would come, even when you can't see a better day, and you can't get over, well don't despair you should get over one fine day. You wait and see.

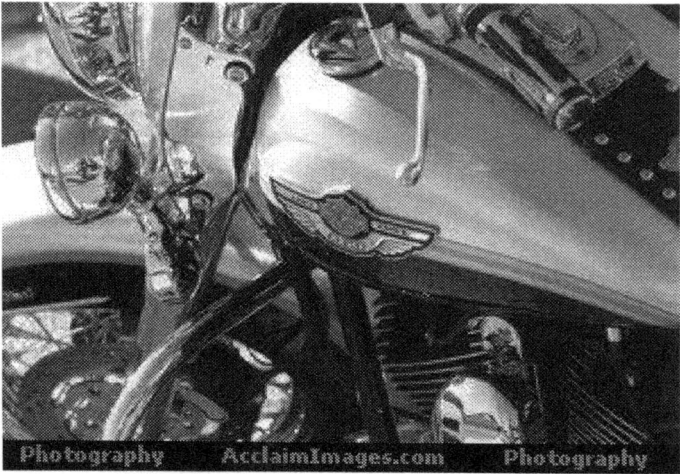
Photography AcclaimImages.com Photography

What you say, see it my way says the male rider as he rides past on the Harley Davidson, what a sight to see, with the wind in their hair. What a sight to see, it makes you feel you on a motor bike with your hair blowing wild and free, travelling at one hundred miles an hour, but don't you think they could be much more handsome if they grow dreadlocks and then get on their motor bike.

I don't mind if it means locks or straight hair, but I think dread locks is more, then again the girl could not be secure with a dread riding a Harley so he'd shave his head sometimes for his girl to feel that he would not leave her for another girl, dread locks would be a gift.

Better to keep your girl rather than to blow the fuse fusion for a quiet life without dreadlocks, and I know if they don't grow dreadlocks they would always be there for the ex-wife or ex-girlfriend and if they had dreadlocks their ex-wife or ex-girlfriend would not stand a chance of getting them back. I might get a Harley and go surfing the road.

When I get my Harley and go on it, it can be just like I am in a play, go for long rides and then come home to play music with the smell of incense and what good Hells Angels do.
The pie and mash shop was just open for an hour and look how many people is standing in the queue. It was a long queue going far back two shops.

Now then I said move up I said to one of the guys in the queue, so I said to myself that I would not wait in the queue anymore. So I left the pie and mash shop, even though I wanted the pie and mash. At first I thought of going to a cafe, where I can have something to eat. That day I went home and made some fry up and that satisfied me.

Now don't sit on a stool and look me in the eyes, and tell me the honest truth do you think I need a man as I am a man or do you not know. That is a question I would like answers to.

Now look at a load of cows in a field and answer me if you were a bull and you was in a field with cows how many bulls would you want, of course one same with humans.

That's why I am not gay. Fair enough if you are gay, it's up to you. I am married to a girl, we are happy. Don't you they say I am sick, well could

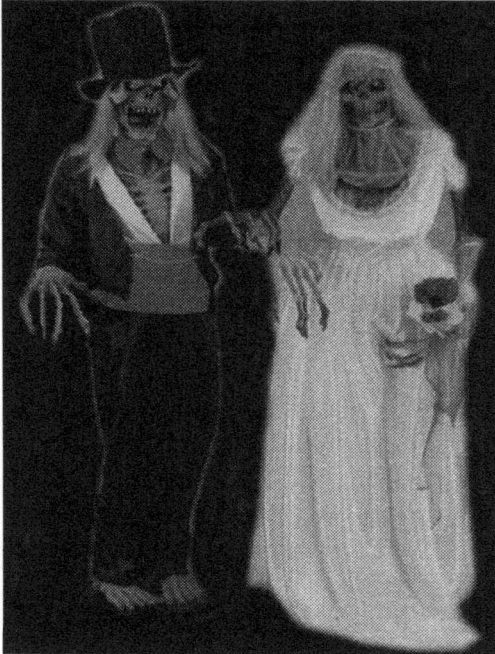

you believe the bad things what you hear about me, maybe a bit of a rebel and it's not that they took the time to look me over. It's because they don't know, they or me, are jealous of me.

Right now I am a bit mixed up and I am getting used to it anyway. I would say I am kind and they take advantage of my generosity. They got to know me as scared but I am not scared and do not pay them when they ask me for money, I just give it to them anyway. Sometimes a guy may say you look like you are his uncle and so and so, well that is jealously talking. But I am not a stranger, and I think you know why.

Hey you know no one answers prayers, then why do you? There are so many reasons why so many people go to church, if you could never know.

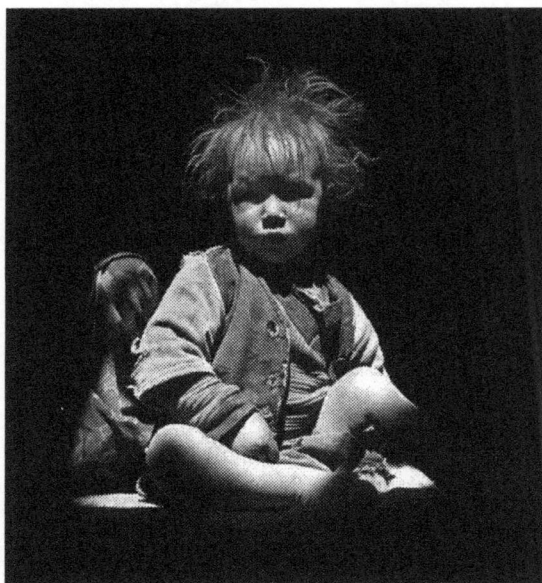

Some people would kill for religion, some people think it is important to go to church and pray, no one answers prayers. Make sure you don't go astray and turn into a fool, for church is for the collection money. You may be a Christian today and a Rasta man tomorrow or a Muslim. How many people would think I am a little bit religious, well it is not a bit. I think it is so.

Listen now son take these few dollars and sit it out, I don't mind how long you can stay when you come back and you can have some more money, and when you are ready to go just go but keep in touch, and you don't even have to thank me.

When I was growing up, money really mattered. Now I know what it means but look how much money can buy, money is the most, but I am generous with it anyway. Now as you see there are lots of mixed marriages and if you don't know you must be part or leave it so the children can have too.

Some say it is fashionable; they used to say I was dirty because of the long hair, but we know it was cool. There must be a better day, why would you have to give the few dollars back. And now a few words about the rise and fall of the so many beast, but not just yet.

This tale has been bugging me, don't say we have to dip it in acid and see if it changes colour right on. All right look now it has always been that way, can't you see there are not lots of misers now.

Just like the baddies has been around for a long time, it looks like the baddies have been there such a long time I call them baddies, spy, beast, cent epée, or worms, call them what you want but you know that they're holding back the younger generation, be there with the rise and fall of the so many beast yeah.

Yo, yo has anyone seen my girl that plays my six-string guitar, are you like that. I should be writing a few lines about the girlfriend, if she has the guitar in tune, how could her favourite songs owe, no not at all, and the way the girl plays me the guitar, how could we owe.

I spend my time trying to remember what we have done, she holds me like a tune, my girl can play guitar good, quite good so we have a lot of times even films [home movie] playing the guitar, and I

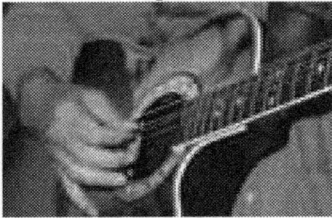

told her that just to have someone that plays the guitar is good that is just a bit of the fun [playing guitar], you can have and let me rock you steady. Your friend the giant, or is it just the way I do my thing. Now look at this, what would you call me if you look through the eyes of love. What would you do if you find out that I am not ten foot tall?

But you tell all your friends how you know a friend who is great and he is good, and he stands ten foot tall. How could you forgive me if you tell all your friends about what you think of me and it did not reach his or her requirement? What, would it break your heart? I have never been let down, but if I were, I think I would be back to put giant back on the map.

Can you see a lot of churches they give thanks and praise and then them get down on to the chapter and pray to their own God or whoever? Now look what that guy is saying you can't pray to that God that one pray to mine, mine is stronger. Look at the morning service how it goes on for a long time, hours and hours and as you leave the church you can forget about it if you want. Now pick some lord Krishna music they would never let you forget it.

Others say if you were a Christian you can forget, just because they would say you are a Christian it would be all right. But if you say you are a Jew or Islam they would not forgive, peace and love has come to them, yes they can have their blessing from me and I know they should be blessed. Yet you have your rights to do what you would want, not that they should, not even Christian you should not have a God. Why should they have a God?

Look how religion cost lives in the World War II. It is always the Christians that complain, why must this be, check it out. No one should have a God that kind of thing is old fashioned.

The nice times begin with a three course meal in the evening now watch this space for it is not the only one like that, even though they always say it is the worst it is not the first one like that, but in these days of mass production you can't say it is the worst.

Now I have won at least an Easter egg at Easter with a little voice saying you have no Easter egg without Easter bunny. No fast and dirty play, to tell me not to do what I want to do.

From the alleyway to Buckingham Palace, from the park to Broadway can you dig that kind of talk as they say you should know?

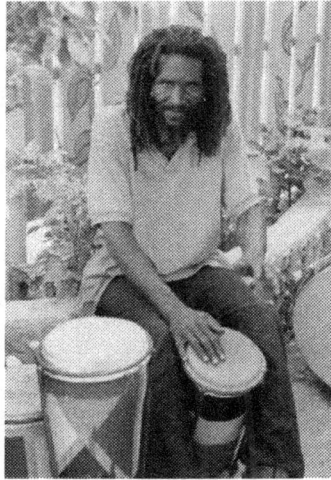

Yet some of them look at a pot and say you can't cook some even have a pose to say you don't eat eh. Why should you sing in the alleyway, why from the smooth to the rough and rough to the smooth? When can you score on the brand new remote control circuit, so everyone has one and I say you should have one also, if you want you must pay the price, not pay the price like a crook must pay the price, but in a nice way. That was something mother would cook.

There is many ways to score if it's not clothes its hats but you must score and have a good time coz these times are good. No one that you know should get it wrong. Look at that day it was just an ordinary day, just like the day before just an ordinary day, why would someone want to spoil an ordinary day. Well that is how it is them that try and get in the way, see if they won, oh no.

For there have little tolerance for spoils so take the phone off the hook and just chill out? Yes, yes can you hear that music in your head pounding after last night session; even if you are black or you are white you can enjoy the nice sounds. There was a sect call the Skinhead they were white that was way back in the 1960's they liked the reggae.

The Skinhead adores the reggae music; you would think they were amongst the first fans of that kind of music. Did the skinhead worship Jah, no one knows but they love the reggae, they must have come after the Rasta's and to this day they are the biggest buyer of reggae music, wasn't they cool, to see another sect like them rise like a rebel of these days.

Room service for the new sect five star hotels. If you are staying long, I just said lots of nice things about where I live. There you are nice big bunch of roses, but there is no vase to put the roses, wait she said, I am going to get a vase.

This place is just an intersection to you, this place is only until you find some place else. But I don't like this place much it gives me the creeps, and you know this place was just to keep me from being lonely. I know what I am doing here and I might get to get used to it with room service and lots of good meals and a telly.

When you see me write word like Skinhead I am not winding up anyone, but for instance, natty dread was known to be for the smooth and not the same as how it used to be. So keep saying the Commies are coming or how people of the past used to say long after the war, they used to say the Germans are coming. So now they looked at me when I had dread locks the same and it is better to leave those kinds of ways behind coz they should be forgotten. Big up the new generation of dread locks.

May they find a better luck than what the ones of the past saw filled with peace and love and lots of money. Something I should have is to have a service, good girls to come and visit me, after all it's only a few quid, but it is better than going into a bar and buy a drink and not be sure you can bring the girl home so be sure. But be sure to use a condom yes.

Don't you think it is better to wear a condom? I always wear a condom for those kinds of girls, can't you guess that those kinds of girls are not always nice.

Now where are you going this time of the night they say the shop opens till late, sometimes all night, but you know the shop has lots of crowds and they might mug me, yes even for an ice cream. So what are you saying now you are a nerve of mine?

You say you are really close, I said true coz you are really close to me, I said when I feel like I am cracking up I turn to you. Some of them say I am mad some say I am generous but you really knows me, you seems to know what I am doing, Look the wife she is really good, she get all my jokes, we are close, and no folk, yes, no folk can say we are not close.

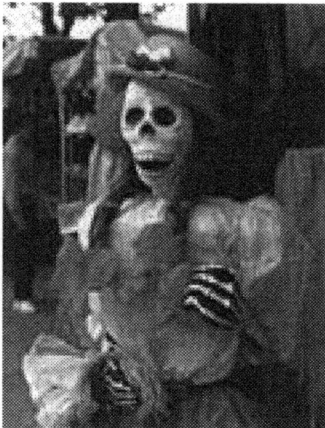

Do you think you are well known, if so hear this, I said to a lady that just comes to town? I said let us go to the bar and have a pint, she said what is a pint? But one pint of beer, I did not know it exists, it was not to drink one larger but it was what it is. So you think you are popular well you may not be as popular as they think they are. Hey somebody said to me why are you so grey [my hair it meant] I said that is the beginning of the good life, and because I have lots of fun and lots of other fun and laughs.

The reason why I said that is because they were taking the piss. Could it be a fact, I said to myself, I'm not even worn out, anyway. Me and my grey hair it must be that life only start when you begun to have grey hair and I have said it's when you have lots of children and it is when you feel sixteen.

They say life began at forty, look at the children growing up to be a quick forty coz they say life begin at forty. It has come. Let's join the revolution of the rebel. Now look at all those people that forget how quick fashion goes out of style, most of the kids growing up will become yuppie that is they get rich then we have the miser who never spend any money but who are rich.

What we need is to let them grow independent without exploits. Can you use the wrong force to let the kids grow up properly?

You can say and I know you should win now looking at who they are, and they are strong and they are the force for the future.

The thank you revolution should start thinking thank you, but you don't have to lick no arse. The last tune played as the crowd disperse, the sound of the cars in the street is so quiet and the smell of petrol and fumes is just too much.

All that fumes if you strike a match 5-1 it would blow up. Those days were the good days for the best tune, and there was not a single fight and the girl looked so sexy. Hey you why not take a cab to get home. Oh yes I take the mini cab; it won't be long before we can get home and to bed. The four of us laughing and whispering in the back seat of the cab as we are going back home where we live, later it rained and you could hear the rain falling on the street, this was usually winter time. But the reason why I go to the dance is to pick up girls when I said the girls was nicer that not saying the girls are not just as sexy because they are just as nice. But it's so nice in some of the clubs, better known as the disco or now they call it house.

Do you know that walking on the crack on the pavement is not bad, it is just a superstition and what about walking under a ladder that was one too, and there are so many superstitions?

 Well I make it my business to try most of the superstition but I had to pack it up and go. As long as you know that I call the tune, here I am again, they know that they are all right, fire away, which means call your tune I am a good listener.

We can find and cover any day one day after the other, and I am sure they would be at the start of the next day. Just like it never went, I told them I have looked at it and it was perfect now watch them come and pretend they never saw me repair it and every time I repaired it they say they never saw.

Do you know they never saw, right because I was in charge, I say it is just because I am in charge they said they never saw. The next day I went to a bookie and placed two bets and waited until the race has been run. The first and the second came in second.

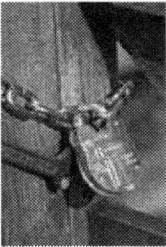

Oh how I wish I had put the money each way then I would have got back my money, so I said to myself I might have been lucky if I put it on the dogs. I must say I am sick and tired losing on the dogs or the horses, but sometimes I win anyway. The reason why there are so many prisons is open and empty; some of the crimes are so petty that they don't have to go to jail. The same criminal that got off for petty crimes go on to do crimes again. Listening to the television the other day I said to myself why not buy a car so I could get to far away places and save on the fares.

That was just like a dream, now I won some

money I have no wants about getting a car. Now I am looking through endless magazines looking for something to do. Why should you stop your boasting and pretending, boasting and pretending that we are without limits, and there is nothing we can't do?

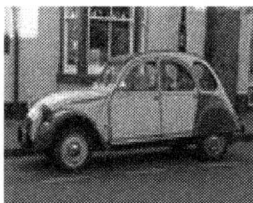

So it's like no tolerance, which is something I would like to do in style of the best of a hundred things to do and try and make it more fun. But there has to have a tolerance even if it 7 percent, there has to be a tolerance. Could you play marbles like school boys and do small boys take driving course, no, when you could be getting into the groove, of which is no ones business but for ours. The few that remain should see who not in the groove as it is hooked on a groove, a rock and roll grove or any tune you would like to play. Trespassers will be prosecuted, so we must be off the plot in two weeks.

Which are two allotments, each allotment could only grow enough food for two weeks. If you know what you want you could grow anything. Some things are worth much more, so it depends on what you grow. As they say about the English weather anything you want you can grow, there is nothing you can't grow. I grow tomatoes the best ones, look how the food that is grown in allotment is much better quality than what is on a big farm.

There you go again about you are born to be wild
and lapped up the freeness, does that mean that
someone would sort you out by knocking you to
the floor, that means you don't have to be wild to
say you were born to be wild. Most kids are wild
anyway, does that mean I am a fool, no quite the
opposite because I am more than new clothes,
and anyway could I keep up with new clothes and
the fashion, even though you would like it but as
these clothes come into fashion soon after it goes
out of fashion again. About wild, wild, wilder than
wild if you don't know, it comes in like a rebel. I
have always had the fashion of the day.

Come on, that's foul play, oh you can't do that,
after all you seek a cowboy. Try it as you see it.
You are too deep, try and stay on the road and
not too slow on the road. Stop the car and let's go
for a walk for a while look at them just going far as
far as a mile away. Sit and rest in the car before
going back on our journey.

Right from the top to the very last drop and so
and so on, the bass came in like my bass guitar
player which we call moon bass, when he plays
bass guitar its like you are in the guitar, with moon
bass playing everything is alright.

A perfect day to see how moon bass learnt to
play, he had to learn to play it from a long time

now. I know what moon bass can say is I got the sweet music in me, and know that the radio is the best, for music. And now there are many photos of third generation slap and tickle or bump and cream, to create like new, to live like John Williams, with the third generation umbrella, and shoes, while selling T. Shirts so I could unblock the road. You would think the guy was rich with on his shirt that has been ironed out, yes moon bass was rich.

The money was a lot, he had a car only one owner but for piece of mind he had lots of fans, and played his own guitar.

They were so jealous about it because it was not a gamble to own, and they were all winners. They were really good and when the guy could not own they went on like they could do it also. He could not make my girls even when he was a big star, my girls stuck to me, like the leaves on a tree.

They could not learn my song, but this was not boasting and toasting and pretending, and laughing and grinning that it was five but they could not own my ways, some but not all. Grin some purpose or don't grin at all, when you drive your big car and you see me on my bike you laugh but you did know that I only use the bike for exercise.

When I am in my car would you see me as I ride a

bike, try and adjust to what you see or you would be out to see is alright with me because you are like me and I know you would like to be like me anyway sometimes.

Same when I tell my jokes you said you would want my jokes, can't you see my fans are laughing, and you say you can't remember my jokes and you want more of what you can't so that is not cool.

I know my jokes are good jokes but guess what, someone said they must stop me laughing because I laugh too much.

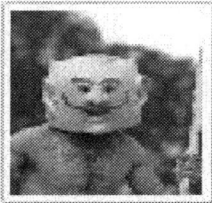

Then there are those that say I never laugh even when they know I do. Big up my jokes. But I don't always joke; as you know coz I have lots of work to do anyway. Now come let's see what is best for us in and out of good times and bad times, and have a lot of good times, look where you go even though you have no need to fear coz I am into the good times and the bad times also.

Yes look how nice we are together sometimes, isn't it so. But I don't always laugh most of the time I am cool and nice just like any other citizens I have so much for you, you could call me brother.

One bad apple doesn't spoil the branch. There is always a baddie in every gang and don't you want it perfect how it should be, I want it to be good in and out of good and bad times, but really I want it to be more good than bad, take the, rough with smooth.

Middle weight quiz player, climbing mountain I think the way I am thinking now even Mount Everest is not enough for me, reason, reason, reason why Mount Everest is not enough for me, is it's like when they win the Olympic gold and you are proud then, you want to climb to a higher heights, like climbing Mount Everest it makes you feel so good. But to my best is my best and you know you should not try and do more than your best. But it is close, but I would like to be much healthier, but they say I am wise and not play the fool when I am not to.

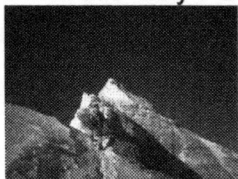

Who am I, well I am a man with a drink problem, and sometimes I go to the bookie and spend hours trying to win some money, spending my time up the bookie but not mad well not as yet.

Well today I have a horse that could not lose and don't you know the more I bet the more they lose. One day when my horse come in so does the money, coz it is so. Every now and again I become a drop out, and then back on my feet but

I am not a down and out, right now I am a drop out that's right.

I am not a down and out so I will get back on my feet, but gambling does not make it any better. If you are too rough you can't know me but I have always say take the rough with the smooth, now for the last few days it has become almost impossible to do anything.

But last night I was looking back at that I got on after budgeting heaven knows how I got all that money in my coat pocket and how it went so quickly, next time I must save and make my money last I got it to save money so one day I can have what I want to buy.

I had to say to myself look how much it would cost and if it is more don't buy it, try and budget the money coz time could be really rough. After yesterday and today after all I done they still wanted more what a greedy somebody, what a pig you mean to say you mean you see, after they took all my silver and beg for more. Well I have stopped begging down the street where I play the guitar but it was fun anyway.

Today in two hours time I shall be going to see the football match at half past two. Well I not jealous of the team that is playing my team, but you see their kit was is such bright colours that you wouldn't know what to do with their little colours.

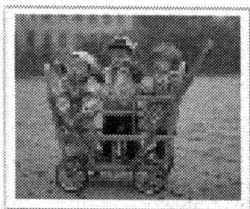

But I shall still go even though I would like to see our team dress like them anyway. I have not seen them play football as yet but I have heard lots about them, even their socks are bright so I am pissed off, never mind. But its same type of football team, the two of them, I won't be bothered to go to see them play anymore, but for a while I would keep their team photo on the wall anyway.

Why do you go around like you are Peter Pan said the wife about her dad but she has to be more kinder than just trying to wind him up, so much of that and a bit like Peter Pan.

But she did not know that Peter Pan stays as a child forever, he is not a child or think like but she says he looks like Peter Pan. But now I will call my dad the same name but I hope the wife doesn't hear me for there is nothing nicer than to be called Peter Pan.

Now we shall go drinking with two girls, after drinking we will take them back home, but we have been waiting for an hour for them to come, but look at the time. They won't be coming again it's kind of late, but don't worry about them two they wasn't a rock anyway.

About this is the last time I would talk to those two girls, do you know how they look, they look like they stand up men every day, they was not a rock anyway. Look how much drink cost anyway and there is no guarantee you would get a bit.

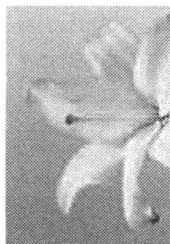

It would be much easier if you do business with a girl prostitute and you would still have change from twenty pound note so I am glad they did not turn up but my mate said he wanted someone clean to spend the night with. Always wear a condom, you might say that I am cheap because I pay for it but that's just sometimes.

The day they read it, it was to say he was more than me, but the few always try and bluff like they could win. Just a few of what you call the opposite colour and opposite sex, but that's all we would need for this moment, they were not rare but there, though they were more but really they were beggar who found luck.

They had a convincing smile but you could not thrust them because they had a sore and had to pretend they was still up on top and laughing. But they came and thus it's not the same as joke but they were like the Mormon.

Here we go again they say you are the ringleader

and also an ex-pimp, but they also say when in Rome do as the Romans do.

Oh yes oh yes how come you got the time if you did find the time and if you did not have then somebody else would have.

You can say you had many cars but that's not much to me, what is yours is yours and I am sure I have more than you. You may say you have everything but I know that I have too.

That's not much because you can't go to the nearest star, so stop showing off like you are better than me, coz you are not. Now you are waiting for the new type of radio or television, see if I am jealous of such things, no way. As they say Rome was not built in a day. If it's hair then it was food now its clothes, what it could be next. Horny no he said a wee bit horny.

First he said he does not know where and could be jealous as I said first it is hair then it is food, are you crazy just go to your own house and get your puppets to show you the way I said coz I know I could never paint you and leave you with my brushes and I could give you more for a better day, when I say for a better day I mean don't add any more to their lice and scales, and dandruff. They say knowledge will increase, we all limp but we must try and get it together coz we are close and have to do more than the do, so far we don't know much but soon knowledge should increase then we could have and know what we want.

Soon we would start to know just the virgin earth, we would learn more as they say knowledge would increase, some people will find out more but look how it has gone, look how one sided it was, with one nation finding every thing, or the rise and fall of one nation, or could be more, I can see lots of peace and love.

While the dance is over, well what would you do, must go to dance to be the captain of the rhythm, watch how those lights go round on the disco floor.

Well now don't you see the disco lights is a big deal coz it's quite pretty. I have both on the beach and on the sea to look at the fishes in the sea and there is food for so many, there must be something you saw, why such greed could come from the sand, do you think it is worth fighting over.

Oh yes look at it close and look at again, don't you think it could it could be better, if the time is now. Look at what I am saying. You may say get over the blooming bad weather and after there are many nice places to go and even if there are not such we are 100 percent perfect.

Yes he did not do it, we have to help him out, yes

lads, on compassionate grounds, all it was, was a sweet and bitter incident. It was so small that we had to let it go, you could just tear it off and forget it.

Love told in a far away land that is including the languages and cultures, new folks with their new food and drink.

They said long time ago they were told not to speak; for the land was conquered by a conqueror that was long time ago they were told not to speak because that would not suit their conquest.

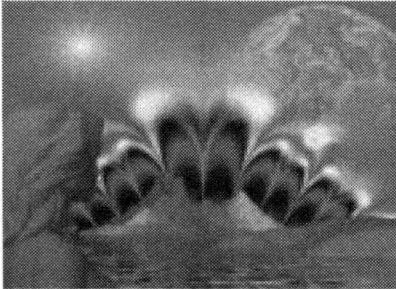

They were told that it was crazy how they dress, so when they look at hippies or Rasta's they say that is not new, but it has not been around a long time now, just something that reoccur all the time through history on and off, but they found they did not want to change everything.

I don't really know but the cavaliers hair style looks like, was it like dread locks, or was it curls if it curls maybe it would be tangle up coz really I don't think they could afford to keep their hair in the same condition for as long as the style lasted, that would be too expensive. But the time says we have lots to do and must be moving to do something else.

At least the Punjabi kept their turban for hundreds of years anyway. Everyday I say it is today Monday or it is today Tuesday or whatever the day is, it is time to be moving to something new, so hold your head up, because we can see a revolution for the new. New rebel of the day, but a rebel has to be a good rebel to survive.

They say if you can't get it right on time this time then you would get it right another time, so make space for the new. So hit it right on the nose, and try and see if you can make it like it has to go.

Now look how the tune has been called, and the wind of change has been called or is to be called. The way it is looking, it beginning to look like harmony and is not far away like a sculpture, or the way the river rode the bank and it has to happen.

The new gipsy that has just moved into town, they collect more junk than what the church jumble sale, but had good aims. That is why we have to say peace and love to them. Not that I ever heard of those sorts of people, but they are always rich, and they change, so how can they get richer? As far as I known those kinds of people has been around for years and they could never do a thing that they don't want to do, so I saw the gipsy, so it is.

Then again they don't make much trouble so they could stay in their own community without being in the way. I wonder if the gypsy always says about people like me. I wonder if they say the grass is always greener over there.

That is what they say or sometimes close to what they collect. But this is not rubbish. But it is what they are used to. But I know what they want. But I say it has to be good anyway.

What a bit more, they say you can't be certain but I know you can and so and so, they say there are coming with things what you don't want to know, but what they are coming with is so nice that you would want to know anyway.

I have what they don't have, just like transistor, deflection, as so much radiation in your personal computer anyway.

To start it is like a three course meal looking so cool but it is not love, so it is like a piece of soap which you wanted to hear but jokes can't fill your stomach. To know what I mean try and be kind, think of them as a capacitor spacer if they lose.

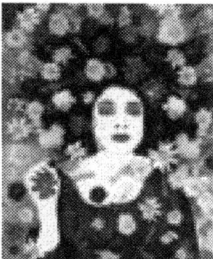

Don't you think you should be

getting tool for the damages caused by what someone done if they came to upset you? Or if they must be thrown out on compassionate ground was it done so that they could not harm.

Well all those with tools for what you did not know, you should get a grant to pay for the loss of what they had. Now there you are saying they only pick on you because you were soft and they though you were scared, as they found you were not scared see how quick they run come with tools and money.

Now they want to give you gifts and how many past times to full the gap of the day, and you're so big up with your day and your pastimes. All right what is wrong with them then, some of them say they are laid about not doing a single thing all day.

Now watch how the day goes by with lots of things to do like the sand [so many reasons]. Now it looks like they don't even have enough time to have a bath. I call them drop out, some call them schizophrenia, but it wasn't always what the doctors used to write on the doctors records, you know what they used to do, well it was just like slang's, such as "wocha" and many other slang.

Look at what that the doctors had back in the nineteen seventies; they used to have this craze of calling every visit mental disorder. Ten years later they started writing that it is schizophrenia, and then the nineties the craze started to go crazy about stress.

I have a few ideas of what it could do in the twenty first century, but I won't say. Flares are back and I wonder how long would it be before they bring back mental disorder? The smokes were more in those days, but still in contact with what is going on with them anyway. I wonder which doctors' records would make the best smokes, coz they all have their trance.

All you need to do is keep yourself clean, just by keeping your clothes clean and they can't call you a schizophrenic that can't be bad... I only have an hour before the good exam and it is very important for me to recover once again and show that it is possible to win.

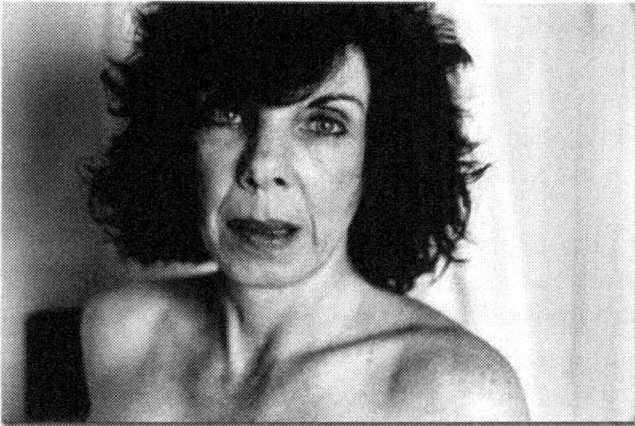

The rise and fall of a drop out and rise again and the rise and fall of schizophrenia and rise again and how they recover. But it is easy with a little touch, like when we were small our parent said keep clean so I am saying maybe wash behind your ears.

To get over is just a little soap and water and all would be well. I wonder how many suffragettes there is in town, that I know, well I don't really know but I think it is a lot and what about how much a suffragette could make in a day begging? Some say they don't have to beg for long, what you would get in two days work.

But if you live with something, which could be anything for a long time, it becomes a way of life.

Well I say me oh yes, I have had many nervous

breakdowns, and that sometimes it is one after the other so many rises and fall and back up again.

Well I have fallen in and out of love many times before, so I have, so it is.

Look how everything is going all right now. Sometimes I look and I can say I don't know how I survive and it is not just saying that because it is a fact.

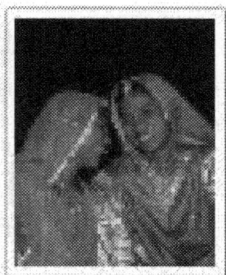

Sometimes I think of just picking up what I own and go somewhere else where I can live better yes, yes sure. They say the street of Japan is paved with gold, or there is milk and honey somewhere else. Oh how I wish it were so.

Right now my day is beginning to come together, but most of all the grove that is in style is getting more and more like how it is supposed to be. That's not too bad, now look at how many times I said I deserved more, so look how much I would go for a happy ending, peace and love.

Now look at how someone that I can write with says they could be good for me. But its not that I am giving up the wife coz she is great, but I need a lot more than what I have. But not more than she can offer coz I want what she has to offer.

This is not just Dick Whittington pantomime, it is for real. There must be a way to find, and even when it is close which it is, what I want so watch me now. Just like some of us can find, well I do think that I can find also but not right this moment at this moment. All I could say it was lies too good to be true, it could never work I did not know the girl too long and she said slow down a bit and we can make it work for us.

The same girl that said I should slow down and looks at it like it was new. Now it looks like I could never even remember her as she turned and walked away but I would try anyway yes, I must concentrate so I can remember her, because look how many times she said she love me.

But it is looking like greed, all these ladies loving me, and now I don't know which one of them I want the most, but all is all I think I would pick the wife. But I don't know which one I would need the most. If I had to forget one I don't think I could force a smile or even have a drink.

Look now, look at how many times I pass all I know is that, I must be much nicer coz I say, "hello, how are you" and try my best to be nice. I just don't know how long this "hello, how are you" is going to last, coz you are more than just a 'hello friend'.

You don't know how I try to be more of a man or a girl, each day I am always smiling to greet you but all I can push from my lips is, "hello, alright?" and walk on pass you without a little sentiment to show how it should be.

I know it is all right but must get on better to be perfect. But this is not what is meant to be, but I must try harder, and make it more perfect for my 'hello friends' and me.

Maybe next time I could say come with me to my home and make my day.

I must make an effort to be much more, here we are rubbing shoulders and now we pass each other, I must try and bring her back to my place where we could have lots of fun. Maybe this time I could nudge, I am sure I can nudge it this time, but this time the same happens, I am sure this time I will nudge it this time.

Don't wrong me when you know that I am right, I said to one of my friend's and I said to the friend don't take my kindness and say it is weakness. When I give that does not mean I am scared, I said. You must have a reason for coming to see me and don't try and spoil my day. I had to pose my fact and that and I don't always have to pose. It is like you never heard a word I said or don't you take notice of what I say.

There were a few guys I use to know we got close and after all we did, did not look like my work or even cheer me on when I was winning. Instead they loved me as though I never needed more than fresh air, but that is not what it is.

And another mate of mine, he knew that I went to his town sometimes so he stayed where he would see me come into town, just a friend that came every day so he would not miss me if I came into town.

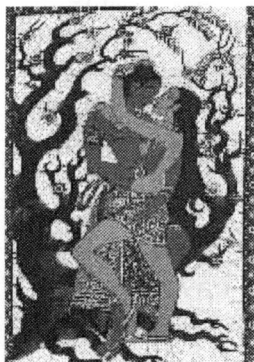

That is not the answer coz I had more than ordinary love, I have lots of love addiction. So when I did something for them they were never grateful and they would not appreciate what they and I done wanted it for love, and not even as much as that.

I say I wish they would not take my kindness and say that I did not mean that. Even though we made love regularly, I can say I get high on your love, she once said what kind of wanker I was. She said that she could satisfy me and I would not need anyone else, but I know that is not right, a man always needs more than what he can get and even more so I told her just because I am with that does not mean I don't want.

I was not talking to her for the sake of talking. I know that I need that girl but not so much, that she would be the only one for me.

Someone only say that when they want to take me for a fool. It was like I was in turmoil in my head with me thinking weird thoughts, I should do this and I should do that, I found these days I might always remember. But some of the days are a long time ago.

But music kept playing in my head, and a little voice said you don't have to take that anymore. But the music playing in my head kept on even when they heard that, it was enough. Sometimes it is because the recording is not the original and the recording is not as good.

So what I did, I said if you carry on like that, like you are more than me, you would have to stay smelly, so try and get the best recording and it would be ten times better to have a better recording. I was not supposed to be in prison coz you are not so hard up that you can't get the best music.

I thought it would be over by now but instead you kept on looking for something that happened years ago.

Well sometimes I have a bad day and sometimes

no one upsets my day and I say to myself you can come back and everything will be all right again and look at the one that had tormented me.

But that is a long time ago and I am just looking back, that is how I know how I must do without people like that. I can live without enemies. So if is so and you want more of what happened a long time ago, don't you think you would start to smell or go bald, that I said to the man but what he said he likes his spot, and would rather go bald or smell? I said if you think that is good, you think it is good but move on, that you must. More wine.

I think that I could find better ways of getting my kicks, maybe let the side of my hair stay long and shave the top, or go to the gym and work on how to get the ultimate power exercise to make my arms stronger.

I know I could go and exercise and get my self to an ultimate fitness for that is what I might want to keep fit. And don't forget to throw out all those; what you might call empty bags that have no use to me.

The other day I was so lonely even though it was just for a day, and I did not even look for one of my friends, I just thought I would see how far it would go before someone visit me, why? Because it is always me that usually make the first move.

There it goes again about that day. I planned
what to do if I ever had a sad day again, now I
could never have a sad day again for I have
sorted that out. Well I am saying I sorted that out,
you know what I mean, just sitting looking how it
was looking at all those plums kept me from going
insane even if it for just one day at a time.

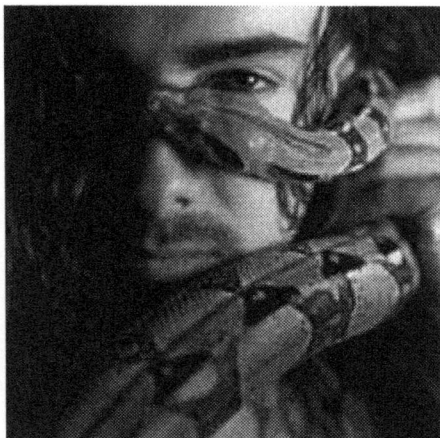

At least I know
how to stay busy,
and I know I can
do what I like,
don't you know I
feel just like disc
jockey doing
their own thing.

My mate always
says think big
when you are
under the
spotlight and don't let your friends get you down,
or they are friends but not some of them on a bad
day.

I say I have to learn all the tricks of what is in at
this time, all right the new trick. It would make a
lot of people happy if you look good or at least try.

Think big as you should know that you are the
one, the most, the way you make me laugh, I told

the wife but it not all laughs, but it is time. You must realize it is not always fun being married, I must say you give me that extra push and say that I am a wise man, who is very important anyway.

It is always her to put it right. I am not saying a man is no good well he knows all the short cuts, but it was not a game coz she knows just as much sometimes. But there is one thing that I don't do is right wrongs. So it does not matter if they are men or woman, I always have to stand up first, it is not anything because I am just saying we are the same type of people. I must have said that lots of times and it is so.

Now can you come to tell me that I am so important, that if I say a joke then you would look at it like I am more so she should listen to me, if she did not I would be lost, I have to tell the guy that it was not a joke all the time, but she would always get my joke because she has a good sense of humour, and we are lovers, so.

Now don't you think you can have lots of fun [laughing] and make it your place to be there, coz you are a mate, and when it is your turn you would see if you don't look like me. Look I am like what you except to see as I quote from one of them song just sowing the seeds of harmony, and I am that.

The HIPPIE MUSEUM

Peace Love and Learning

Don't you see how I am writing peace and love
and if it is not peace and love it is the best quality.
Here it is again it is peace and love not crime, no I
don't like crime. If it does not suit you to see
someone speak out on how to stop these crimes,
coz crime makes someone's life unpleasant.
There is no way can someone say this is not who
or what.

Look how I know how long I have known what
and who's, what I have been around for a long
time now and even had many good jobs. But right
I have had fault finders saying this can't be you,
yes it is I, they say you are next to nature John
and have nothing to worry about. It is something
like that I have in my mind, just like the seasons
and how the wheat grows so nice and the rain
falls so sweet on the rooftop.
So am I to smooth out the wrongs that goes
through my day and that is a lot of work, and I
always say I have a lot of tolerance. All this is in
a days work. Yes some people just like you to

spend all because you have the money, these kind of people are very mean, and not worth much, they would like you to spend more than what you have so you would beg them, A big, big up for peace and love, nice up your life.

Here we are again, when is a door not a door, well we have to go through that again and that the tenth time today.

Here you go again but this time with a little more serious plan, look how these laws keep me going and going with a perfect stance, but with no progress.

Maybe enough of that and now I am able to find, and look in through the past for mistakes so I could correct what I done in the past few years, and for the future.

So I have to look through my past coz I have done so much and I done lots of things like the sand, when I say just like the sand I mean so many reasons, it is to build a better future.

So I have to find a better circuit round about linking the past with the future so we can add and subtract plans for the future. Now try and find a grove and keep that grove and be as you are to make a better day, isn't that what we are looking for, to make a better day for you, me and whoever, so we could add to the past lessons and

you could stand in the future and make everything
strong.

As one of my laws says husband and wife should
share so the wife can be just like a lighthouse
shining all around the rocks, and lots of acquired
attitude to lead the way for a better future.

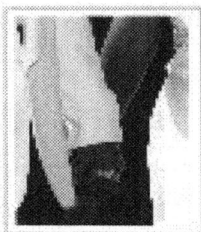

There is a bond between
husband and wife and now try
and be a little flexible with what
you do, with a bit of give and
take, it is not give and give, we
have to stand firm that we don't
fall apart.

Yes we have to. Oh no why did I leave her for
another girl coz really she was quite nice but at
first she was that kind of girl that would see fault
in little things such as spitting as something really
bad and would keep malice and the kind of
woman that say no and always say sorry when
she did not hear.

But I can forgive, but sometimes it is so ridiculous
but also quite innocent, but there was no reason
to go on like that.

Then after a while she stopped all those bad
habits and started to be more like me, but some
people say you can't change even with a long
time to practice, they say you can train a dog but

some people you know you could not really change.

People that can't change should not be with a wedding or someone should really put them in their place.

She was not the type of girl who had no tenderness because she had; those people that have not a bit of tenderness but a bit like when they talk to you would wish they would put a sock in their mouth to shut them up.

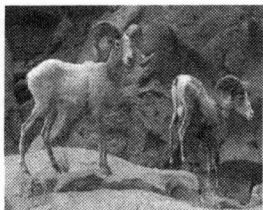

I am so glad that I got over those kind of people, you can spot them just by talking to them for a few minutes and you know that they should be nice and have respect.

Even thought they were failing their parents' footsteps and they say such thing as pardon instead of just saying what, and they would like to know why you said what.

Do you know that there are people that find fault with nearly everything? Some of us do and don't know what they are going to the next day and they don't think they are going to do that sometimes in the future.

Look at that man chewing those kind of chewing stick, but who know you could pick up the habit and start chewing those chewing sticks, now look at that man saying he would never do it and start to make trouble.

Who has the right to do something like that after we are big and have been living a long time and go on like they have no experience in how other people live but they want to complain and get in the way of the young, and people that try and please the young.

These men that say you can't do that can't find and are very fussy and have to change if they want to be good with other people.
Are you the heaviest and does that mean you have more sense, alright let us go fishing and if you look you can hear someone saying [calling a bluff] fishing is a quarrel sport and you should mind you don't go fishing no more.

Such things exist if you don't know, as you are going to do something which is good for you, and then someone come and say don't do it, [because it might make you too big for them].

Oh look it so, look at that one just walk past look at me look at that stare and it was to put me off my course, and now he looks back again like he is saying you could do better.

Now what is it you are going to do now, as I said there are some of them wishing you bad luck as they are saying bless you even that you know they are trying to spoil your plan.

Here you are again been nosey, well you don't have to look there, when they can look somewhere else so what's the hassle, why there I said don't you know that if the girl look there again, can't you leave that, that did not do me justice. I think I more a lot more so why would you look at the same tale over and over unless you dig.

I am just saying you must stop it I said to her, now don't look back now o.k. coz I have done so much in this time and again it does not make justice. How could they be so unkind? So try and be careful and don't be sad, you don't have to cry, I said coz every one that I know they can make mistakes, so don't look at it as bad.

If you were bad you would not have got so far. Suppose you call someone a really bad name such as black nigger and you apologise a few times and give some money to charity and even try and be friendly with blacks. Would you forget those words black nigger [or even white bastard]?

If you did all that a friendship would have to follow, a bit like Robin Hood of Sherwood, how they fought on the bridge, and then they became best of friends. That could have been a Skinhead at Stanford Bridge too.

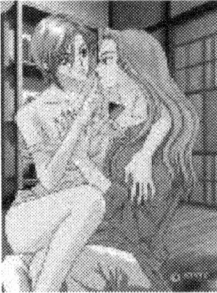

Now they are saying the seven seals are flashing and the night at the bright light zone was where it's at.

Do you know what, that woman was made for woman- kind, that she knew what was selling. But what the men had been piss, but I am saying it is the wrong time for these women to act like men. You are too late to be a man and they had to throw those out because they were too old to change now and after all they were womankind, just like they wanted to be the opposite sex. But I said it is too late to be a man, so you have to learn all the nice things to keep you staying a woman.

I said she has to wake up and be a woman or even putting it nicer to be a mother.

From a long time ago they told of one day they will see three brothers, which was worth much more than fame. But they don't know what or when it will be as the tale went on to be known lots of woman were cutting their wrist and saying this is the seven seals.

This was a day they said for these days are the days plenty and yet to come, but the three brothers kept close to each other even though they had disagreement but they were close to women.

Each one of these was so perfect and cool that those women found them perfect and if they did any wrongs the women would hide what they did wrong and their shame.

The woman accept them as their friends, a bit like Wonder Woman but these three brothers kept out of the way of other men and select only to have women friends. That was a story a girl told me about the three brothers then it became a sect of men that had problem with men so anyway you hear of their names or the story that means you want a rest from men company. The three brothers were cool anyway, but that was just a feeling they had and found out that that was a bit childish, everything turned out all right and they learned to share their food with both men and woman. They were happy to get over the little hangs ups they had.

Then there are some people without values would see something is o.k. and they find little faults like there is something wrong with it or there are some people that break something to pieces like it belongs to even more because it does not belong to them.

And again some people start something and when someone said they are cleverer than them, they say they can do it better like writing or singing. They said they could do it better but they could not do better without you showing them what to do.

Sometimes they even copy you and then say their copy is better than the one that put all that work into the original, so some of them steal ideas and get you to smash yours because they were jealous of your good work.

They go on like that because you are from the same kind of working class kind of family. They try not to pay you for your work, and they never see where you did good and even if they do they would not give you the credit you deserve.

Some of those people would rather smash the work instead of paying for it.

They would smash it to pieces and then you can't find it again and they think that is better than you having whatever.

Sometimes I look at electricity and think was it like how they smash other peoples work to bits, was it suppose to be a whole city and somebody smashed it to electricity as we know it today. Bet it was electric food and clothes or anything you wanted when the first guy started it. I bet the first guy that made electricity someone told him that they would kill him so he smash it to just a light. That means they smash the sum and now no one could put it together again, a bit like Moses smashing the Ten Commandments.

According to my probe can you remember in the news when that guy said he had a breakthrough so that we could live to be two hundred years well I think that is what happened to them.

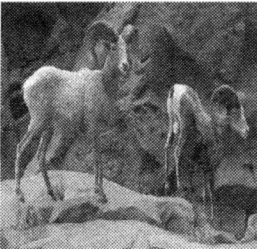

As far as I know they were told that as soon as they finished it someone would kill them, so they did not do it because they thought that the people that tried did not deserve it. They said now that we know how to do it they would kill them so all the kings horses and all the kings men couldn't put it back together again… for a few hundred years.

I just meant to say that I am not getting in your way, but it was like a block of stone and it was not worth much. That's why it was just stone, but say it was made of precious metal like silver or bronze or even more expensive metal it would be worth a lot more, but it was just stone.

The steps I meant that's what I said when someone said ' I wonder how much it would cost to make three flights of stairs', I said thoughtfully it may never be worth anything in the future, but stone steps is what we use and steps are not usually expensive anyway. I said to them, they first make the stairs out of stone and if you want you could change it later, so to think that you can put off some things for a later date would make you want to do a lot of putting off things that you should do now.

So try not to put off some things that you want to do if you could afford to get it done.

Watch that man, one on the left now, hear what he said he would never be there, well what I said at least he knows, and then he began to stare and you know they saw.

Now look at that in a court house or just someone who said they saw, do you know that you would be seen too as an offender if you do the time to think about it, so when you know and is pushed into your corner and they you did more to stare than to say it just as guilty if you know and did not say as to do crime.

Feel no way about what you wanted as children is now what you can get easier than those days, there is a lot you can get free, and what I like most of all is the way they are giving away free

c.d. in most of the news paper and the magazine
they give away looks so expensive.

Look how the mags would cost when they are full
colour. Look how much it would cost in the
twentieth century. But now we are in the twentieth
first century, and we can start to look out for lots
more changes in this century but one thing I
would not like is a something like a war because
look at these days it is peace and love.
But look how all the other century there has
always been war but this time we can feel safe
with the United Nation, it looks like there could be
no war and the future looks secured coz we
should look after each others and keep
peace and make sure if there is a conflict it would
have to stop coz we have to keep peace coz we
are more civilized than what they used to be in
the past few centuries, not like the little war in
Iraq.

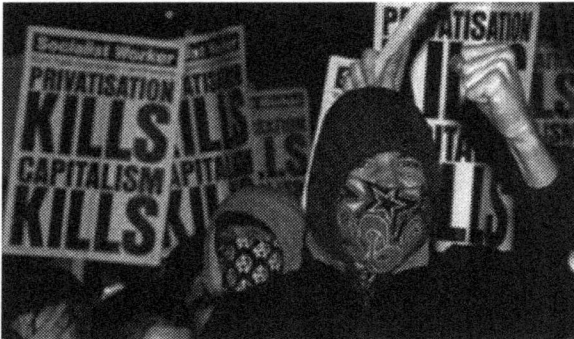

Let us learn to live with each other in these days of freeness, and in school they should teach the children what we did not learn, and I think there should be no adult singers singing to children under sixteen.

The songs that we heard in the past should be done by children for children, a bit like the J.5. and really young singers doing their own thing to some of the classics of the last century.

Then you could be proud to hear these kids singing instead of hearing these hulks for men singing for the children. And then they would not have to look up at big hunks singing to them and they would be more independent and it would help them to be the ones that do their own thing.

As I always say, see how much you can use your judgment for what you are doing and you should be all right.

I know that every time you do something and if it goes wrong more than once, next you should know from your own judgement not to do your best until you are sure. Then you could whatever and when you are sure you can do it you can blow the fuse [go full out].

And it is important what you call, don't put all your eggs in one basket, but how many people nowadays would know about eggs and baskets, so to see much save in two accounts, try and do every things in twos, so when disaster strike it would not be all lost.

That is something that's always bothers me so I am doing it that way so that I don't have to lose.

We know we can't keep living that way, no we just can't live like that so now we have all our eggs in more than one basket so that we couldn't lose, because some of us have been losing for such a long time, and it should not be that way.

But now that we have got that sorted out because we are not all winners in what we do and have to make less mistakes like that those people that are losers do.

So it is very important not to make the same mistakes, we have to draw a line if you are going to lose, try and split it so you don't lose all.

A good way to remember is a scale which would balance so both sides is the same, same to share what you do and not to do too much, but quality is what makes you keep your standard, but don't put all you eggs in one basket, I think it is so.

My mates always say think big when you are under a spotlight and don't let your friends get you down.

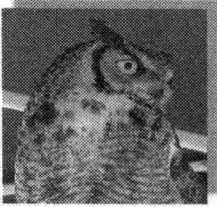

I say that I have to learn all the trick of the trade, all right the new tricks.

You could make a lot of people happy if you look good or even if you can't look good at least you could try.

Think big and you should let others know that you are somewhere near and that you can do almost anything anyway.

The way you make me laugh but don't you know you don't make me laugh all the time but even the end product is always equal to what you put in and can you realize it is not just fun and you could put extra push to say if you are a wise man.

They said only a few of us would know but if you know how to put it right then most of us would know. I did not realize till much later what she said but it was not a game and she even knew it sometimes more than me.

But I said can't you see that you are somebody too, even though you were wrong sometimes, but you were very good at taking short cut.

I said by the way you are going you should have been somebody great, but there is lots of time and what that was, was is now, and you see it could work for you if you could just keep cool and all could be alright.

I hear you saying 'what can I do to let you decide ', I said carry on you little potter, coz a potter is always there to make new objects and I know it could be just like what you would want.

I said to the potter 'you just come with me and we can decide a little later just to see what you would want to make for me'. Sometimes these potter guys can do a lot of pottery you don't want or they don't even want themselves.

Me doing this pottery is beginning to become a bit of a joke, soon as you make something and you want to make something else then it becomes harder and harder to find what to make the next time and pottery is no joke. Did I have to tell them what it said and then would they come back to haunt me, I said 'tell me but not those things you told me they are supposed to be secrets'. You know secrets you are not to tell everything you know.

If you know how to have good fun never mind, if it is in school or at work you can have lots of fun without being to funny. If you are going to have fun make sure that you are there because some people might not want to laugh so to stop the risk of embarrassment try not to make too any jokes.

Don't you think that it is right to have lots of fun but mind how you go, because there are a lot of people that these days would like to fix your face because you might think you are too clever or just that they think you are taking their place and they might not like that, but just say you are a mate and when it is your time I would laugh.

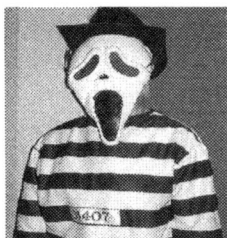

Now I have been in the same situation for such a long time, I don't think I would ever change, well I could get older as I go through life. But maybe in time I should change my ways but so far I am not ready to change my ways.

My prospect is so clear and there is nothing in the way. It is like after many change in the past if I change right now, it would be the wrong move at this moment and it is like years to come I won't need to change coz there is nothing going wrong for me right now.

We all make mistakes and I know I have made a lot of mistakes and I know as I go through life I am bound to make more, but so far I have not made so many really. I don't think I am the worst.

You can call me a strong man, in your defence and I don't know what you would like to call me. Maybe you can't count all yours but don't worry it can't be all that bad coz you are not still not the worst.

Look how this is, they said thoughts is faster than the speed of light and now look at this as we know as we are watching our television you know some alien could be watching our television with us by tuning to our mind, but I think they are primitive like they have a box of plants and they are waiting for it to grow into a television, where there are bows and arrows.

This girl that I knew died a few years ago, before she died she said she would be my probe to see what it was like to be dead. She was only 23 years old, and as soon as she was dead I thought she was going to the other dead but instead of that I heard them say it is John's girl and she has to get the best room in the dead world, she told of how it was and the future but that is just a small department of mine.

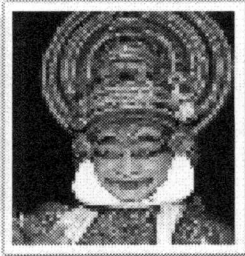

She was very usefully as my diplomat. Later she said she was my dead angel of John who is I who has to look into the future and that she would carry my flag. But after a few years I did not hear from her for a few months, so I told my other girl friend call Kim B. what had happen and I think should go and repair Angela and make her warm.

There she went just like a space man space walking outside of the voyager space ship to fix my diplomat. So there was Kim gone dead to find Angela, when Kim got there she send back news that Angela was in [her grave watching some of those plays that is what the dead do just lay there watching films] an experiment to put a Mask on them and send them back from the dead but the experiment is still in its early stage. Kim and Angela had to go to school to get more knowledge to return; now there were two and they could not find any fresh eggs.

The two of them could repair each other and do my works and she made crosses for our entire problem carrying my flag John of revelation in the Bible.

She said 'John you have something to do the resurrection', and she was not cold rice.

Yeah man if you are listening to one of those songs and you said that you don't like it then you really could sing it yourself and give the one who sang it before the money or you should not complain.

Why I said if you don' like the reggae sing it your own way. I suppose you could do it a little better, coz when I sing I said to these rouge trying to say don't buy that one don't buy this, what I would say to them maybe you can do it better and if you can do it and it could sell a million and we could split the money but don't find fault so don't complain with just say it is good or you do it.

But if you distort someone's work you should pay for it.

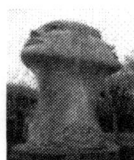

Now we are married now let us forget anything that is wrong coz there can't be anything wrong between us now.

As I put this ring on your finger and look the bride in her eyes then you know that is where it's at, so marriage is where it's at as long as you love the girl. So as long as you love your girl then take the plunge, yes when you fall in love with the girl, marry the girl, or is it that love grows until you find the right time to get wed, and if you don't get married you could lose the girl and someone would married her and you would lose your woman.

They say marriage is down right and if they get married it might only end in divorce, but it is best to let it last a long time.

Then after I got married one day I made a joke to the wife about getting me a girl friend and she was cool and I have not looked back.

To my dad Jude, 'if you not the one, well how does the sun shine. If you are not the one, then how do your shoes fit? If you are the chosen one, well is the fire so bright'.
You can't fake a picture so that's how I know he is salvation.

You sit in a warm and pleasant seat, they say you are the lost elder waiting to be found, my dear Jude these few words cannot tell your name, you are like a moist lips in the desert, peace and love maybe ahead of his time.

This time we have to make plans of what we had and the way to put down the same ones that made me have to put down that good place. At this time because we put down the main plans that we needed the first time and now they have distorted what we had, or is it all we had so we can't start again.

Seen as they distorted those documents we have to look through all those scraps coz that's all they left us with. So we have to use the scrap material of what we had left over to try and repair and try to get it like new.

Then we have to pick out the ones that they had made spoils and get someone that is right for the job.

Now that can't be so easy that would make you uneasy to lie back so it can't be so easy. But don't just lay back and take it like you don't have to work, I say you have to be busy like a light house, shining your light all around and learn to guide those little ones through the rocks, like a little light house.

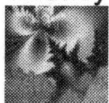

We are the ones that make dames and lords; we are the little worker that helps instead of getting in the way, now put your stuff in public view, in the shop window. Watch those goods go as those people are buying more like they are doing piecework but this is buying instead of working. Look how quick those items clear out of the shop window, at this rate we will be out of work. It can't be just a fixed rate and make sure that you get the right rate for a days work. You know you have to get a lot of money.

But there I am working hard without breaks and enough, but that's years ago, and now I am getting a good rate the soft pieces but it has been so long I have been getting the crust.

They say you can't take peace and love in these days of not so many peaces and love anymore. But I wonder how in the world, meaning they said you could never make it as a hit or you are too bad meaning a bad, bad boy [or man], but this badness was not against the law. It is what someone says and as for whoever or me they said it about.   '

You could get many hate mails, who knows if it is on the internet or just in our minds; it wasn't always smooth as I say, take the smooth road if that is o.k.

They say we have ironed out all the rough and we are left with the smooth and that is how it used to be, but also take the rough with the smooth too.

I have to look good coz we won't always be the ethnic minority, but where you can look into the future, for the past also has a lesson and now we are there into the future and the future is in our hands.
*
These days of sure you are right and you are all right just to be there, but you must be much more.

Look and say we are not sure if we would make the big day and like the three men that went into the fire and got out, so when it is us we have to be sure about the road you take for the future.

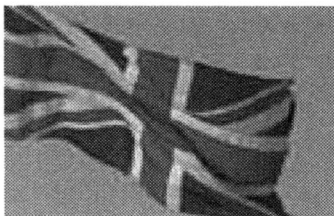
Look at me talking about I have a better road for the future with lots of

look in from the past and peeping in to the future and trying to make no mistake, that would cause us to fall, for someone to say why can't you be trusted.

But I always want your trust as I long to know that you have nothing holding you back, so they can't say you are weak even though you are weak. But why would you let someone look at the same configuration of mistakes, with plans for building a better future and make sure that you know the sum of your junior, and show one step at a time.

There are lots that we can learn from the past, but really that is a lot because all that you could learn from the past there is so much lies coz the past is full with lies.

Assault is one thing that I can't stand and you know. How it comes about even when they claim and some of them claim there is no clues after they assault you.

You mean put them away in solitary confinement, especially the ones that plague on people in their heads, which I call mental assault.

They that are there to give you a bad name and the ones that make you speak out to say you lose your head, and just them been in your head makes them feel like they are bigger but they never last long they always because they are in your head and they are a part of what they put in your head so they miss something and goes mad.

Why would they come when you are having sex? That must be that they are missing that too.

Mental assault can be so unkind when they plague you, when the voice's won't stop, not harm you in your head sometimes for a long time and sometimes they mostly want to boss you around.

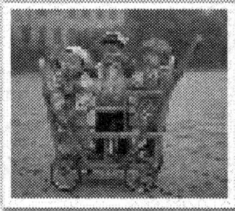

So you would tell the doctor and then he says you are mad.

There are many different voices in head. There are the ones who are sooth-sayer, they are the good ones they would smooth out your problem, and some acts the friendly mum.

Now you must have seen the weed smokers how he says he would give you a hand if the weed goes wrong.

If you can't get what you want but you can have what you need, there is a long gap between want and have but I is so small so some go out looking at fantasy ways like there is always a pot of gold at the end of the rainbow, some try the lottery.

The way some of us try and try and never stop trying coz one found what they want. The day they would get what they want.

But once you find what you would want then you know you are there because that's a start and when you have made a start that is good.

Now you have found it is nice to have a family with a maybe a dog and a couple of cats and you should know what you want coz it is always nice to know that someone who found. And once you found make sure that you don't go and lose it, coz there is a way to find and then there is the same way you find the same way you can lose.

You know when you was a kid growing up, you always wanted to be the star in what you do, wasn't it easy sometimes.

Those days of love were made for the young and those days should never fade away. But really it was hard been a young person as I have just recall, you like to say what you think is right even though the young just say what they want to say sometimes you talk weird and crazy things.

You can't blame the young for what they said and then the clothes they want to wear, the clothes was so good what they wore and keeping up with the smokes.

The wife is always captain but now my friend I call on you so you could be the deputy of what is on the record, and even that you did not sing it sound like you so you be my professor images of those song.

So I said to her don't stray away from the fact that you don't sing but it sound like you, the song on the radio fits you like a glove.

But this is not fame, no this is not fame but the music makes you feel good so maybe one day you would like to sing some of the song that you heard and make the top twenty and you could give the original a part of the money that you get from the sale.

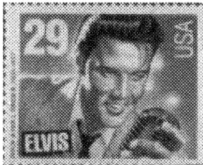

What if you call yourself Bob Marley Jnr and sing all his song a bit like the Elvis look-alike and make them hits just Bob in a style like the Elvis look-alike. Wouldn't it be good a lot of Bob look-alike, but I would say that is too easy for a girl to call her self Bob Morley.

Well if you want to fix the Bob, jigsaw maybe you would give your friend a surprise, I say that is a gift.
I say for a few minutes please stare at me, me John can do without any religion even though I am John so if I can do without but I had a deal at

one time not to leave the religion for most of my friends indulge. If you want religion you can have coz you vote and you can do what you want because you are not a criminal and there is no fault if you try something.

But like most things you have to know when you had enough, because too much of anything is not good for nothing.

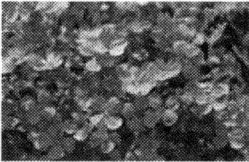

But you see I can act and keep a straight face even when I don't mean it. Put the pieces together and you could make songs of quality.

When some one changes their name I used to why now I think I know, some of these names have been around for such a long time it has lost their purpose.

When you change your name to become a singer or an actor, but they could at least have wanted their Christian name and middle name.

I don't think they could do it for love but they don't so it is their affair but at least squeeze your middle name in. Anyway, names are filled with fun and always summarise and there is no name that is new, well a few.

They say sometimes eh you your name gone but I say, it has not gone, it is just starting.

The Three Musketeers could have been friends without being Gay but that does not matter even if they were, but I know they were good friends, a bit like Rasta man in a one love situation.

They had their motto one for all and all for one, which is like one love.

But how Rasta's live it is a bit like how the musketeers lived and the Rasta's have their own language. Well not language but some words they use as a kind of a Rasta's language and like the musketeers called their friends brethren that's what they us to say too.

I think Rasta men is a good thing for the country because it keeps the nation together, any nation they are in and Rasta man see a Rasta as a Rasta and it is not what colour or race he or she is black or white, Indian or whatever.

They look at each other as brothers and the kindness between Rasta and Rasta is like they are related, even when they speak to each other you can't know if they are black or white without looking closely, and their locks has the same formation, if you see any Rasta black, white, Indian you could not see the difference in their locks, [hair].

There is no difference between Rasta and Rasta; there is like each other, one love. You might say Rasta's why do they have beard.

Well that they are supposed to be if they didn't have beard you might as well cut off the hair off too. There can even be Rasta's without beard coz it says isn't no rules aren't no vows you can do it anyhow.

Then some people would say the hair doesn't look good but course it is all right and I think their locks are nice especially the girls and they can identify with each other.

They are getting to look like each other more and more; yes they are getting to look like family more and more each day.

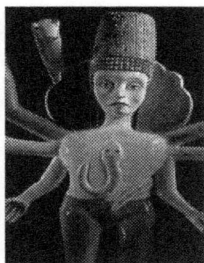

Even if they don't have the religion strong, strong they can bluff and go on like they are strong at their religion, because they are good sport.

Just like a football team fan even if you are not crazy about the team.

When you are with your fellow fans and it is the same with Rasta's, they go on like they are the best and to them they are the best.

Nobody could say if you follow a football team that you are not a good fan, well it is the same with Rasta's and all the Rasta men that I know try and be good. And they have all the gear and they talk as they support it good.

Just like football they have scarves, hats and like a good fan they collect their books as in football they collect the badges and programme every week at football.

So it is not bad been a Rasta coz they have a lot to collect and the standard of life is better than most people because there is so much to do. And that they get the best jobs so it is quite nice.

The musketeers also had a lot too also had long hair. Then there are someone's that say they don't like what you say and how you pray that if they pray. It not that they did not like what you said but they also has friends and without locks for some people it is hard to get on through their days the bald heads black or white.

The ones that do not like Rasta's is a bit like the folks of the Hippies how some people said they did not like the Hippies coz they had long hair.

These are those who keep square company and when they say something about they think it should be heard but they are not the prime minister or anyone, they are just peasants and they don't know any thing about Rasta's, they would say are you a true Rasta man so tell them that you are a fan.

Me, well of all the religion I think the Christian religion is the best but it is not too bad been a Rasta man anyway, so if you usually say it is not a very good religion well it might not be but you can take a deep breath and say it is good.
Some of them use the word Jah only for a toy not meaning anything at all. Most of them never heard of the so called king, but they use it as a toy or just like saying, you are my buddy too and sometimes because you hear it on music and you are a fan and nothing is real they just talk and talk and talk.

Yes it is peace and love too so I am putting some money on my football team to win the cup But I think generous and say you can have many flings as you want and I know that you don't have to be Gay to kiss a man but that would make you one step ahead of your friends.

You don't have to be Gay but maybe doing Gay things is a bit of a rebel even though I am not Gay, I don't think there is anything wrong with it anyway.

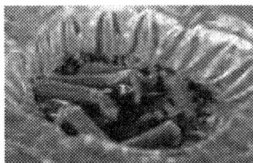

When I was a kid growing up I did not think that I would smoke so I said that one day I know that I could have a gay fling and I would not really say that they are wrong, just like Rasta's you can't say that you are not going to be one, black or white, it is so.

When you find out that you know a bad boy and he did crime, that is not a rebel coz rebel would always be a rebel but bad boys rude boys or just plain wicked is not a rebel, but in case you think I know anyone like that well I try not to know bad boys who would give you a beating for 10p.

So I try not to know anyone like that. But the rebels of these times make sure that you don't mix with bad boys coz that would give us a bad name and so far Rasta's have a good name, they are known to be peace loving people, who try to help those who needs help and it does not matter if you are black or white, Indian or whatever the rebel of our day.

Don't get to be led astray coz you say someone this and someone say that when it is suppose to mean you because you know what and who it meant, but these bad boys are only for a while and I know crime would always be and Rasta's would always keep away from bad boys

So when you see someone doing things that you know that is not what you like it has been told so many times, so just pretend you never saw and they would go away.

But who is good but if you can't be good try and keep on the right path and someone would think you are all right.

Remember the good that you do is what counts, but if you do wrong it is no big thing coz there are lots of poor people and the easier way to stay poor is to do wrong.

When you do good that is when you get other people to notice you because no one wants a layabout, a thief or a bad boy. But once you have crossed over to do wrong it would be hard to come back good, and once you make a name in the wrong circle it would be very hard.

The ones that commit crime are less likely to have children or get married.

Have more tolerance with our friend so we can live in love and harmony with each other. Be flexible.

Everything in the town was going all right; well I could hear some people talking about drinking alcohol, like he did not want his mate to drink too much alcohol. [What I know the wife is my captain Kirk, and we know that marry owe at least two litre, or two pints a week, but you mustn't bring no germ to the wife.]

They were saying I don't want you to keep drinking even if it is champagne.

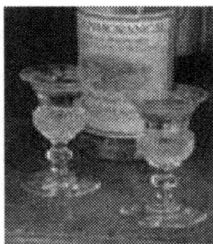

The other chap said that because you can't afford strong drinks and maybe there are a bit expensive anyway. I was saying to myself why would he like to stop his friend from drinking strong drink, there is not much wrong with it. I heard him whisper saying if it was smoking it would be alright, the guy says do you mean cigarettes I stopped those years ago and these days I might start again.

Oh no not just the cigs but the strong smokes like cannabis coz the buzz and they are cheaper than strong drinks. If I smoke they say it is the wrong thing to do and if I drink alcohol it is the wrong thing to do, well what could someone do? They say this is wrong and this is wrong, back to the facts they are so addictive anyway.

Then there the ones that say you should not drink just to make you drink more just because you heard them say you should drink strong drink, and then you have to prove that you are a big man too, which is good, I thought that you would do as they say. I would look at my dad again, the bull of a man Jude bet you thought he was over.

They say he got the fact even before live broadcast on the television, with his little hot legs he is always there with the new, he once said can't you see that I am in the Bible.

So to this day he is respected for his mid-afternoon attitude, for you know Jude is at the end of the Bible where he wrote a letter.

Well dad lived by book of Jude, but he is still flexible because he is still active, sorry but it is so. But I know him, as the real Jude, the one before the end of the book, is it how Jude should be always at the end, and then they catch Jude back in the last book that is the revelation.

Many times I sit with his constructive talk and his plans could bring a better future coz he is well ahead of his time, and isn't that what we would like to hear that he is always there and am glad to be in his company.

I can say why he is not prime minister is that he is well ahead of his time, just like Jules Verne the great writer, or H, G Wells.

So Jules is ahead of his time, sometimes I ask myself if Jules is salvation, they have been known to say the sun would not shine without him, I don't know how that is what and even if they had to wait for a long time they would be waiting for Jules more a bit of the twenty first century he is ahead of the day and for the future.

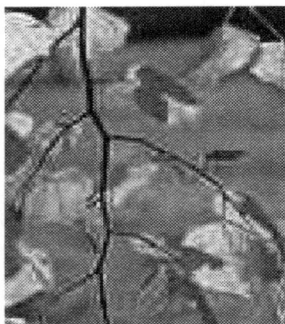

But now it has come to nearly the dusk of his life and I know that he shall be my dad again in the long future for he was a good man, then we could do revelation all over again.

Who know how to win at the races, I am a man that looks investment so I say when there is no other way of getting money, go to the bookie and drown your sorrow by trying to win.

Sometimes you get a long break to win and then you start to lose again. I know after a winning spree you must be careful you don't lose it all back, but the thing about going to the bookie is it is like having a social day out, and if you are a person that don't go out much you would really like it.

Then again don't go to the bookie you may just lose your money, well I go a bit more than once a year but it should be only once a year.

Now I would go to the Rasta man club where Rasta man of all colour go and see if they would help me out with my recording some music maybe they could sort it out for me, coz I heard that their club is quite good.

Let's see what I could do to my music to make it better, now start recording after three. That's one, two, three, this time we can get it perfect just like it should be and this time it would be perfect.

Its one of those recordings that I have to do, but I have to get it perfect so that there are no mistakes.

Now at three we can try again without leaving a gap or a fault on the recording. Even that last time it had a fault on the bass, there were a bit too much bass on it so we have to try once more.

Again after three, one, two three, the selector says that's all right that time, all I can say something that please me is hope it please you too.

Then another time, as it is when you want to buy an item in the shop and can't afford because you are a few pence short not a great deal is it.

Well when you are making a cake you can bake a cake, even if you are a little bit short of the ingredients, but with this little miser you can't have as much fun as you would like to have, and we have had loads of love anyway, so we don't have anyone to answer for or to.

So if you are short of a few coins and they wouldn't let you have it never mind, they are misers and they should never have had a shop.

So big up good shopkeeper. As it is coming to the end of this book I want to say how great it was writing for you to read.

NOW THEN YOU KNOW WHEN YOU PLAY A RECORD AND IT IS SO GOOD YOU WOULD LIKE TO PLAY IT AGAIN! WELL THIS BOOK I DO WRITE FROM THE TOP TO THE BOTTOM AGAIN FROM BEGINNING TO END.

*************************.

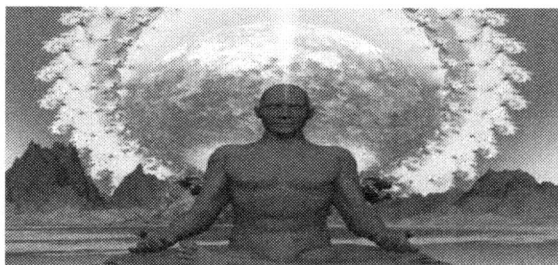